CONTENTS

FOREWORD

It has been said that the British Red Cross Society's century of successful service has been due to five factors: a strong and inspired leadership; a numerous, enthusiastic and well-trained membership; an active and devoted Youth and Junior Red Cross; the support of the medical and nursing professions and the confidence and support of the public.

That the support of professional nurses continues into our second century is ably demonstrated by Miss Louisa Grubb who has written this new Manual for us. Her sound and interesting text, together with the delightful illustrations combine to give us a Manual from which it will be a pleasure to learn and to teach.

Nursing was one of the first services of the Society and the high standard set at the beginning has been maintained ever since. I hope that all Youth and Junior members and their friends will continue in that tradition, for good nursing is the most rewarding of services, giving pleasure to those who practise it as well as to those who receive it.

The Chief Nursing Officer, British Red Cross Society.

INTRODUCTION

Many of you will have thought at some time or another that you would like to be a doctor or a nurse. Instead of waiting until your latter school days when you will be able to choose subjects to study which will help you in your chosen career, you may be anxious to learn as much as you can about looking after ill people now.

Even if you are not someone who wants to study medicine or nursing after you leave school, you will find it very useful to have some knowledge of how to look after not only sick but also disabled and elderly people. It is very likely that one day you will come into contact with illness or old age in your own street or even in your own home; or you may be out walking when a friend sprains her ankle. Whatever help is needed in these circumstances it is a great comfort to people to know that they are with someone who knows what to do and how to do it well. With practice you will find that you are able to make a bed or put on a bandage quickly and neatly and this will give you great satisfaction.

Most people find being ill or incapacitated very boring, so it is important, when you are helping to look after patients, to think of things for them to do. Of course you must enquire first whether they are well enough to play games or make models, or whatever you have in mind. It is also part of good nursing care to do for patients what they cannot do for themselves—whatever it is. For instance, you should see that their flowers are put in water as soon as they arrive, that they receive newspapers and comics promptly, that they are able to reach the wireless or the bedside light switch, that their letters are posted and that they have close to them a drink, their writing materials and book. You will find it helps if you put yourself in the patient's place and think of what you would like if you were ill in bed or could only walk with someone to help you. In this way you will be able to anticipate the patient's needs, and this is one of the attributes of a good nurse.

Nurses must have many qualities to be good nurses, and it is important that you learn to develop some of these.

When you are helping to look after a patient you must be:

1. **Clean and tidy in your person.** Wash your hands frequently, have clean nails, tidy, clean hair and sweet-smelling breath. Your clothes should be suitable for the work, easily washed and kept neat and mended.

2. **Clean and tidy in your work.** All equipment must be clean, conveniently arranged and put away again as soon as it has been used. Dirty utensils may cause infection. Tall containers at the front of a table or tray are easily knocked over and equipment left lying around can lead to accidents.

3. **Reliable** in carrying out the doctor's or nurse's instructions, admitting at once any mistake you have made or care you have forgotten to give so that it can be put right as soon as possible.

4. **Punctual.** Treatment and medicines must always be given at the right time. Because patients get used to a regular routine, they may get upset if meals are late in arriving. You should see that these are ready at the expected time.

5. **Sympathetic and gentle.** All movements should be gentle and carried out in a quiet manner. Talking to the patient in a reassuring voice but, at the same time, being firm with regard to doctor's and nurse's instructions will give the patient confidence.

6. **Patient.** Some people who are sick are not very easy to help; they may be worried, frightened or upset and may take longer to carry out ordinary actions. You must be patient and take time to explain what is happening, what you are going to do or what you wish them to do. You may find that with very old people you have to repeat instructions or explanations several times, and when you are feeding them you must take time and never be in a hurry.

7. **Discreet.** Doctors and nurses never talk about their patients and when you are helping them you must follow their example. This may be difficult sometimes when you are anxious to tell your friends about the work you are doing.

8. **Observant.** You must watch the patient's condition carefully and report any change to the doctor or nurse at once.

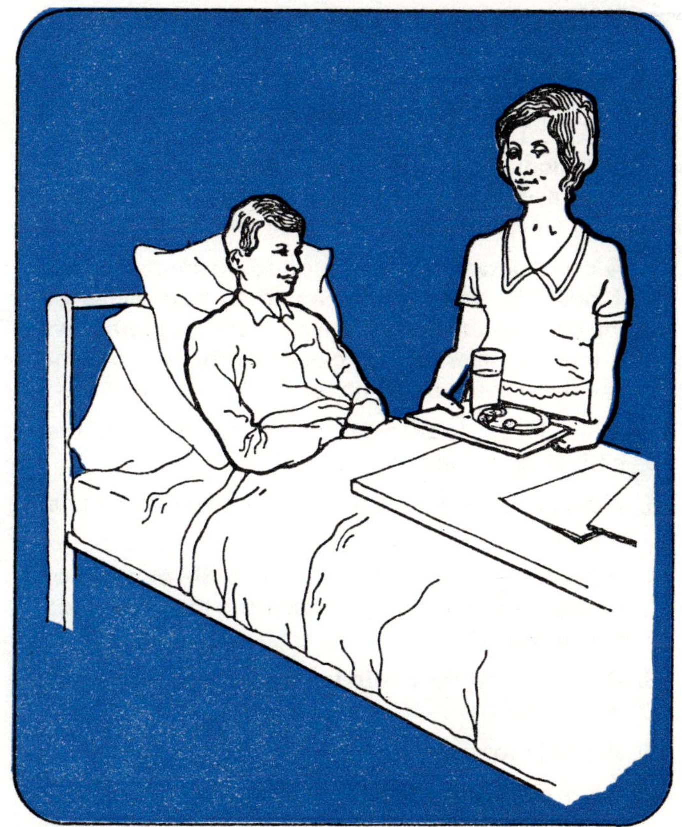

Remember that many people are concerned with helping sick and disabled people. In the United Kingdom the National Health Services and voluntary help available vary in different parts of the country. Information can be obtained at Health Centres, Council Offices and Post Offices as well as in town guide books and libraries.

THE SICKROOM

The room and furniture should be cleaned without raising dust. This can be achieved by using a carpet sweeper, vacuum cleaner or damp mop. Dust methodically all surfaces with a damp cloth. If the patient has a long-term illness, sickroom furniture should include:

1. **A comfortable bed** in a good position so that, if possible, you can get round to both sides of the bed and the patient can see out of the window. A looking glass may be placed so that the patient is able to see what is going on around her.
2. **A bedside locker or table** for articles the patient needs and can reach herself.
3. **A bedside light** — very useful to the patient and the nurse.
4. **A table** or the top of a dressing table or chest of drawers for a working surface for the nurse and her helper.
5. **A comfortable chair** for the patient when she is allowed up.
6. **A chair** for visitors.
7. **Two chairs** for bedmaking (one of which may be the visitor's chair).

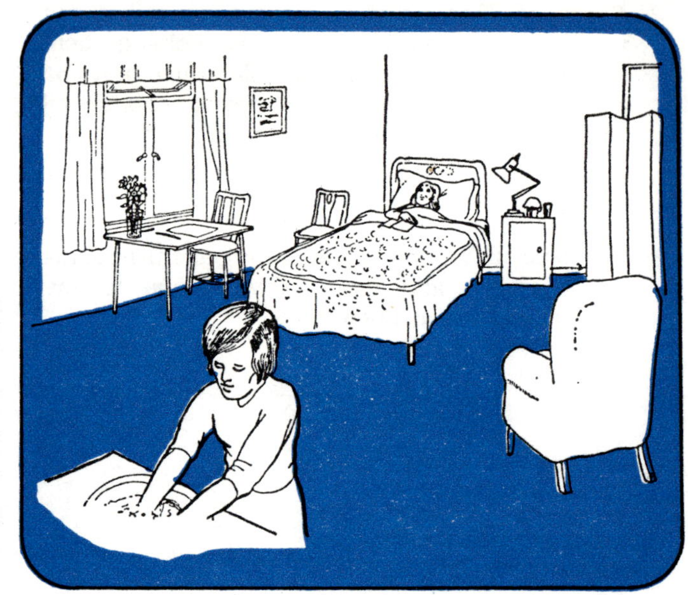

8. **A screen** to protect the patient from draughts and to ensure privacy when carrying out treatment.
9. **A commode** for patients who may get out of bed but are unable to get to the lavatory.

Ventilation

Fresh air is particularly important during illness. A small window may be left open all the time but larger windows should be open for a short period each day depending on the weather.

If there is any draught, the screen, which can be improvised by covering a clothes horse with a large sheet, should be placed between the patient and the window.

Heating

The sick room should be kept at an even temperature of 16°-19°C (60°-65°F) unless other instructions are given by the doctor or nurse.

A fire must be protected by a fire-guard.

Used equipment

All equipment should be removed from the room, cleaned and returned as required.

Meal Trays

As soon as the patient has finished her meal, the tray with all used china and cutlery should be removed. Jugs, cups and glasses should also be taken away as soon as they are finished with.

Flowers

The care of flowers in the bedroom of a sick person is important. It is distressing to a patient to watch flowers die from lack of care or attention because she is unable to attend to them herself.

Trim the ends of flowers and place them in water as soon as they arrive. Take time to arrange them attractively in clean vases as soon as you can. To keep flower water clean stems should be stripped of leaves up to water level. Change the water and remove dead flowers daily.

Most patients like flowers to look at and will appreciate wild flowers you have picked as well as the more "conventional" sick-room flowers. Remember, too, that if it is the time of year when you are able to find very few wild flowers, they can be made into a more interesting arrangement by adding leaves, berries or sprigs of seed pods.

It is as well to remove vases of flowers from the bedroom at night because they are easily knocked over in the dark. Put them in a cool place and return them in clean water in the morning after you have finished cleaning the room.

BEDMAKING

Methods of bedmaking vary according to the condition of the patient and the equipment available. When making a bed, care must be taken not to jar the bed or jerk the mattress to the discomfort of the patient. Conversation should include the patient whenever possible.

To prepare a bed for a patient

Requirements

Mattress
1 under blanket
2 sheets
Pillows — the number according to the position of the patient
Top blankets — as required
Counterpane or bed cover
Eiderdown — if required
1 draw mackintosh } may be required especially
1 drawsheet } if the bed is likely to become wet.

The draw mackintosh should be thick plastic sheeting. The drawsheet should be 1 metre (or 1 yard) in width and 2 metres (or 2 yards) in length. An old sheet folded lengthwise may be used.

Waterproof covers for the mattress and pillows if they are likely to get wet.
2 chairs.

Method

If possible, two people should work together to make a bed.

Cover the mattress with an underblanket, and where necessary, first protect the mattress with the waterproof cover.

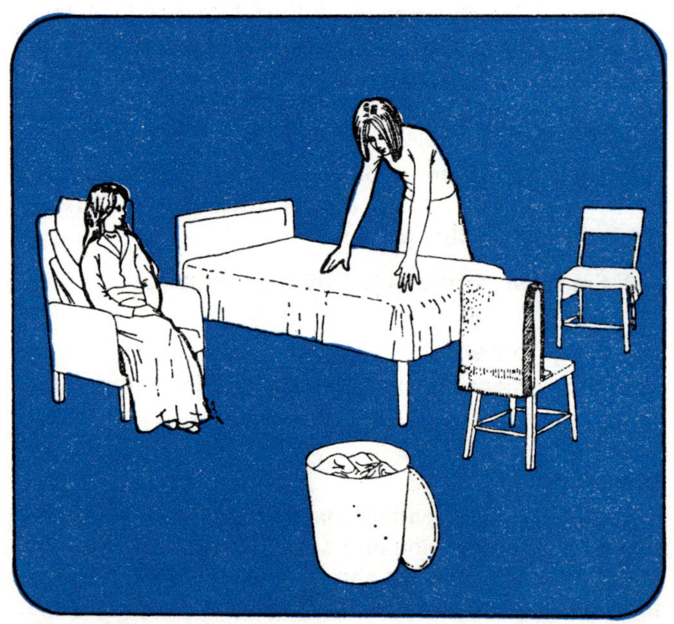

Place the bottom sheet in position, with the right side uppermost and see that the centre crease is in the middle of the bed.

Tuck in the sheet at the head of the bed.

Make square or mitred corners:—

a) Pick up the edge of the sheet about 45 cm (18 in) from the head of the mattress.
b) Tuck in all the sheet which hangs down between your hand and the head of the mattress.
c) Tuck in the side of the sheet.

Pull the bottom sheet taut.

Tuck in the sheet at the foot of the bed and make corners as before.

Pull the sheet taut from side to side and tuck in.

If a draw mackintosh is used place it on the bed so that it will come under the patient's buttocks.

Cover the draw mackintosh with the drawsheet so that one end can be tucked under the mattress and the rest of the sheet can be tucked in on the other side. Draw the excess taut and tuck in under the mattress.

Put pillows into pillowslips, protecting them first with waterproof covers if necessary.

Put the pillows on the bed.

Place the top sheet in position, with the wrong side uppermost, and the centre crease in the middle of the bed; about 45 cm (18 in) of sheet should cover the pillows. Make a pleat in the lower end of the sheet to allow room for the patient's feet.

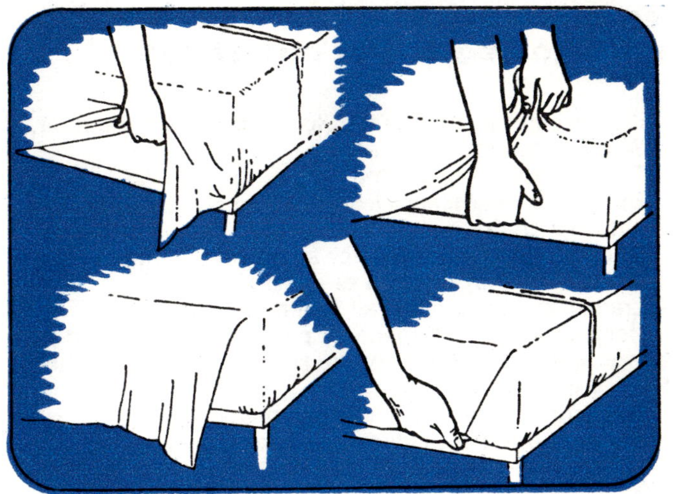

Tuck in the bottom of the sheet and make mitred corners as described above.

Tuck in the sides.

Place each blanket in position, make mitred corners and tuck in.

Place the counterpane on the bed and tuck it under the foot of the mattress; make mitred corners and leave the sides free to hang down. The part of the sheet lying on the pillows is turned down over the blankets and counterpane.

To make a bed when a patient is not allowed to get out of bed

If possible, two people should make the bed together.
See that the room is warm.
Tell the patient what you are going to do.
Bring any necessary clean linen to the bedside and put it on a chair.
Bring a linen bag or bin for any soiled linen.
Place a chair at the foot of the bed.
Loosen the bedclothes all round the mattress.
Remove the counterpane by picking up the top edge, bringing it down to below the bottom of the bed, then folding it back on itself.
Place the counterpane on the chair.
Remove the first blanket in the same way.
Remove the top sheet leaving the patient covered with a blanket.
Fold the sheet and place it on the chair.
Remove all but one of the pillows unless the patient's condition suggests otherwise, i.e. she has difficulty in breathing.
Keeping the patient well covered with the blanket, roll her away from the side of the bed with the excess portion of drawsheet. She must be supported in that position by your colleague.
Brush out any crumbs.
Roll up the excess portion of drawsheet, mackintosh, bottom sheet and blanket to the patient's back.
Tuck in under blanket and sheet again.

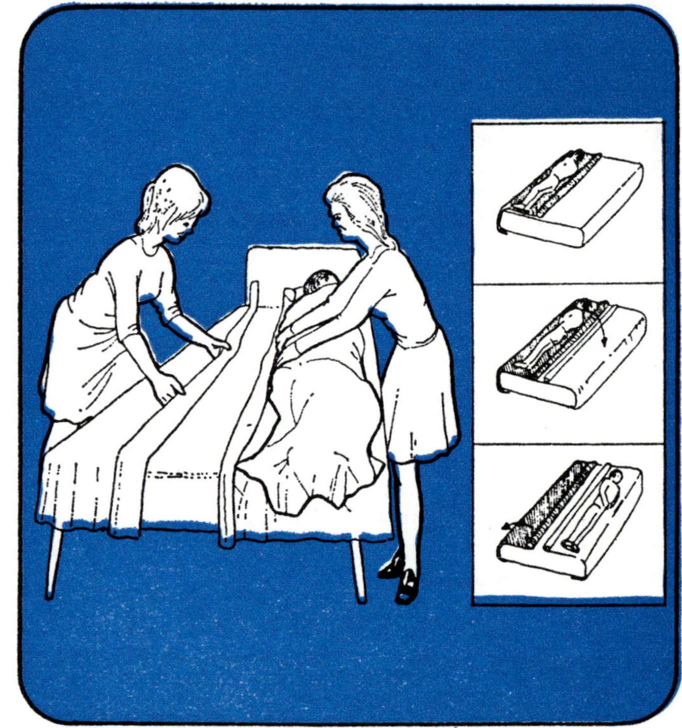

Tuck in the drawsheet.
Roll the patient to the other side of the bed, and attend to the side on which she has been lying.

Make sure that the under sheet, mackintosh and drawsheet are tucked in tightly, so that there are no creases.

Roll the patient back to the middle of the bed.

Pull the mattress up to the head of the bed.

Shake up the pillows and replace them.

Unfold the top sheet over the blanket.

Remove the blanket from under the sheet and put it on the chair.

Tuck in the sheet making a pleat to allow room for the patient's feet. Leave approximately 45 cm (18 in) free to turn over at the top.

Place the blankets over the patient and tuck each one in separately.

Replace the counterpane and turn the top of the sheet down over it.

To change a drawsheet during bedmaking

Tell the patient what you are going to do.

Prepare the clean drawsheet by rolling it up.

When the first side of the bottom of the bed has been made, leave the used drawsheet rolled up close to the patient's back.

Tuck in the clean drawsheet and unroll it until it meets the soiled one.

Roll the patient carefully over both drawsheets.

Remove the used sheet, place it in the linen bag or bin and tuck the clean one into position after the rest of the bottom of the bed has been made.

To change a bottom sheet during bedmaking

Tell the patient what you are going to do.

Strip the top bedclothes and cover the patient with a blanket.

Remove all pillows but one.

Assist the patient to roll away from the side of the bed with the major portion of the drawsheet and support her in this position.

Roll separately the drawsheet, draw mackintosh and bottom sheet the length of the bed up against the patient's back.

Straighten the mattress cover and long mackintosh.

Tuck in the clean bottom sheet at the side, bottom and top, checking that the centre crease will come in the middle of the bed.

Roll the free portion to lie alongside the used bottom sheet.

Unroll the rolled part of the draw mackintosh.

Tuck in the clean drawsheet and roll up the excess.

Turn the patient on to the clean sheets, moving her pillow under her head as you do so.

Support the patient while your colleague removes the used drawsheet, rolls up her half of the draw mackintosh and takes out the used bottom sheet.

She should then unroll the rolled clean sheets and make the second half of the bed.

MOVING A PATIENT

To turn a patient on to her side

Two people are needed to turn a patient; never try to do it alone, unless the patient is very small and light.

You and your colleague should stand either side of the bed.

Strip or loosen the upper bedclothes.

If turning a patient on to her right side — turn her head to the right.

Cross her hands on her chest.

Lift her left leg over the right one.

Standing with your feet apart, roll the patient on to her right side.

Make her comfortable by adjusting the pillow under her cheek, placing her arms in a comfortable position and slightly flexing her upper leg.

To lift a patient

At intervals throughout the day it is necessary to adjust the pillows and the position of your patient.

If it is desirable and possible for her to help herself, the patient does so. She is asked to put her hands on the bed slightly behind her and, bending her knees, to dig her heels into the bed. She should then lift herself whilst you assist with an arm under her axilla. Instruct your patient to drop her head forward and to keep her spine slightly flexed during the lift.

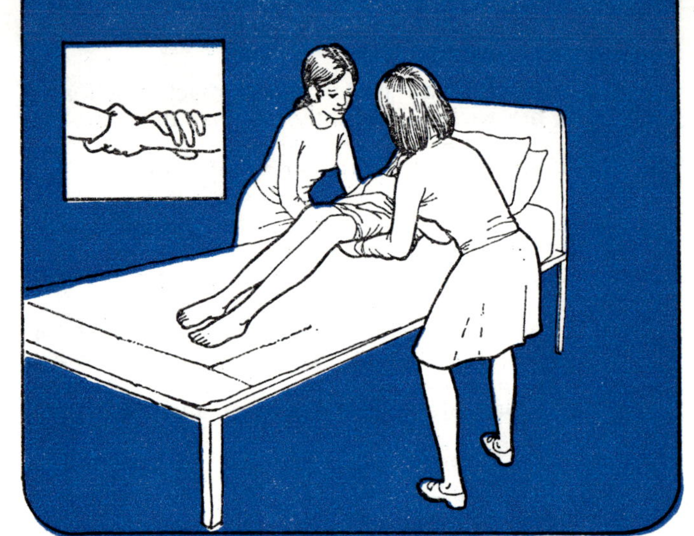

Learning to lift a helpless patient requires patience and some understanding of body mechanics.

To lift a helpless patient who is lying flat and needs to be higher up the bed. You and your colleague should stand each side of the bed with your feet apart and your knees bent. Clasp your colleague's hands under the patient's thighs and shoulders. Lift the patient by keeping your backs straight and allowing the weight to be taken by your thigh muscles. To ensure that you and your colleague lift simultaneously, count aloud — "One, two, three — lift".

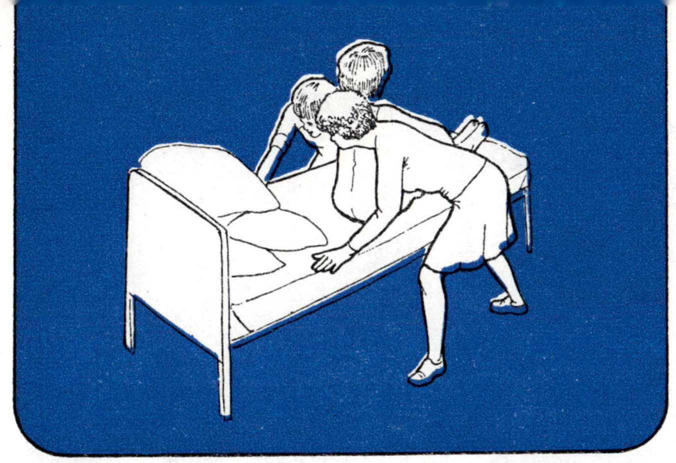

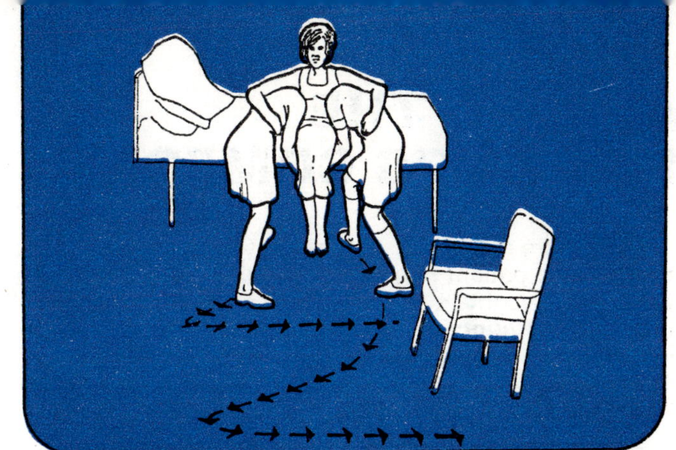

To lift a patient who is sitting and needs help to move higher up the bed. You and your colleague should stand each side of, and facing the head of, the bed with your feet apart, your knees bent and your back kept straight. Clasp the hand of your colleague under the patient's thighs and put your shoulder into the patient's axilla. Ask the patient to rest her arm on your shoulder. Place your hand on the bed behind the patient (or on the bedhead) and lift simultaneously. This is called the Australian method.

To get a patient out of bed

If a patient is confined to bed for long periods, complications such as pressure sores and thrombosis (a clot of blood in the vein) may occur, so whenever possible the patient is got out of bed. It is very important that you ask first whether the patient may get up, and also whether she is allowed to stand or walk.

If she is allowed to sit in a chair, the chair should have an unfolded blanket over the seat and one of the patient's pillows at its back.

Help the patient to swing her legs over the side of the bed. Put on her dressing gown and slippers and assist her into the chair. Fold the blanket round her legs and, if desired, provide a footstool.

If a wheelchair is used, be certain that the brake is on or get your colleague to steady it.

The Australian lift, as described above, can be used to carry your patient to a chair if she is unable to move herself. The illustration shows how you must walk backwards and then forwards at an angle.

AIDS TO THE PATIENT'S COMFORT

There are a number of appliances which can be used to make the patient more comfortable in bed. Some of these can be obtained from Medical Loan Depots of the Local Authority and many are provided by the Red Cross. Some can be improvised. Aids which are used in the bed must never be placed on the floor but on a chair or table to keep them clean.

Pillows Extra pillows are required for a patient nursed in an upright position.

Backrests may be like either a small deck chair or the top part of an armchair. A backrest is placed at the head of the bed and pillows are arranged to keep the patient sitting upright. There are on the market specially shaped pillows which give adequate support and comfort to the patient when sitting up.

Bedcradles are devices used to keep the weight of bedclothes from the feet or legs of a patient, by forming a tent over them. A bedcradle can be improvised by using a stool or a wooden box.

Air or sorbo rings may be used to prevent pressure on the buttocks and wool or foam pads may be used to prevent pressure on heels, elbows and back of head.

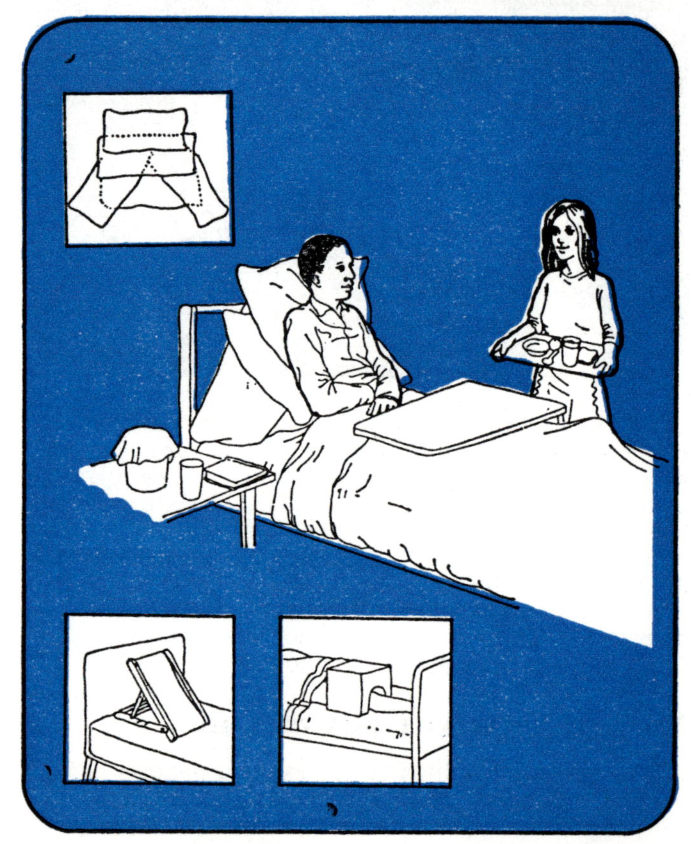

The following aids should only be used after you have asked the nurse or doctor about them

Footrests A bag filled with dry sand and a padded board may be used to support the patient's feet to stop her slipping down the bed. It should be covered by a sheet tucked in under the mattress. If no sandbag is available, a hard pillow may be used.

Bed blocks Wooden blocks are sometimes placed under the legs of the bed to raise one end of the bed. A chair may be used instead but it must be very firm and very strong. Great care must be taken to prevent back strain when lifting a bed and at least three people are needed when raising an occupied bed.

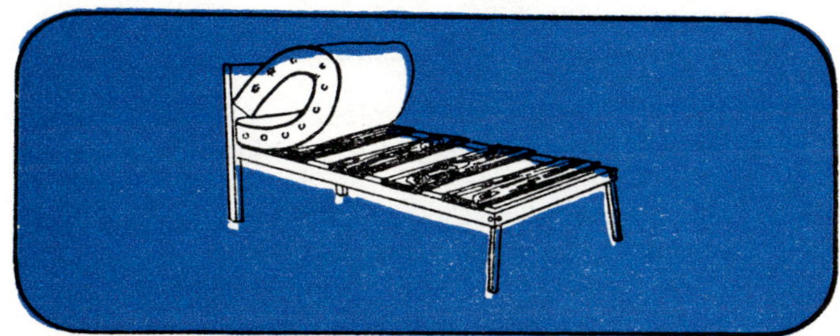

Bed boards Sometimes wooden boards are placed under the mattress to provide a firm surface for the patient, or to provide level support for a broken leg immobilised by a splint or plaster.

Hot water bottles If a patient is given a hot water bottle it should be a rubber one.

To fill a Rubber Hot Water Bottle

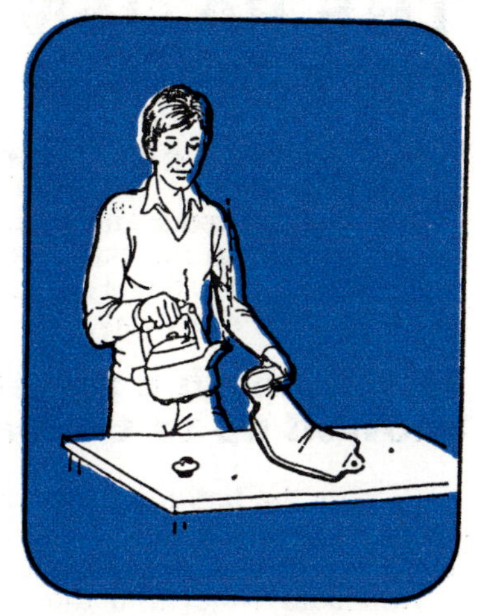

Check to see that it has not perished.

Place it on a flat surface and exclude all air.

Half fill the bottle with hot, but not boiling, water, always using a funnel, if available, to avoid accidents. Make sure air is excluded and put in the stopper securely.

Test for leakage by turning the bottle upside down.

Totally enclose the bottle in a cover before placing it in the patient's bed, with one blanket between it and the patient.

Never put hot water bottles in the bed of a paralysed or unconscious patient. She will not feel the heat and may be burned.

Electric blankets and pads If an electric blanket or pad is used to warm the bed, it is very important to ensure that it does not get wet. Because water is a good conductor of electricity, the patient could receive an electric shock or burn. Follow the maker's instructions.

THE PATIENT'S TOILET

Care of the skin and nails

Sweat evaporates and dries on the skin. Excessive sweat may make the skin sore or cause an unpleasant smell. A patient will feel refreshed if she has a bath or a wash all over every day.

To help bath a patient who is allowed up to the bathroom

Prepare the bathroom first by seeing that the room is warm. See that soap, flannels, towels, talcum powder and clean clothes are in the bathroom.

Run cold water into the bath and then hot water, until the water is a comfortable temperature to the hand.

Some patients can bath themselves but others may need help. Never leave a young or sick child alone in the bath.

Escort the patient to the lavatory first and then to the bathroom.

Give her the opportunity to clean her teeth.

Help the patient to undress, to get into the bath and to wash.

Help her out of the bath. Dry the skin and help her to dress.

Accompany her back to the bedroom and help her into bed.

If necessary, help her to brush and comb her hair.

See that she is comfortable and warm and has anything she needs.

Return to the bathroom and hang up the flannels and towels to dry.

Clear away any other equipment you have used.

Clean the bath and leave the bathroom tidy.

To bath a patient in bed

Find out whether the patient is able to bath herself or needs help.

Tell her what you are going to do.

Prepare all the equipment near the bedside.

Requirements

2 large bath towels to protect the bed
Large bowl water
Jug of hot water } unless there is a washbasin
Pail for used water } in the bedroom
Face flannel
Body flannel
Soap
2 towels
Talcum powder
Clean nightgown or pyjamas
Clean bed linen if indicated
Bag or bin for used linen
Nail brush and scissors
Brush and comb for the hair
Toothbrush, toothpaste and water for cleaning teeth

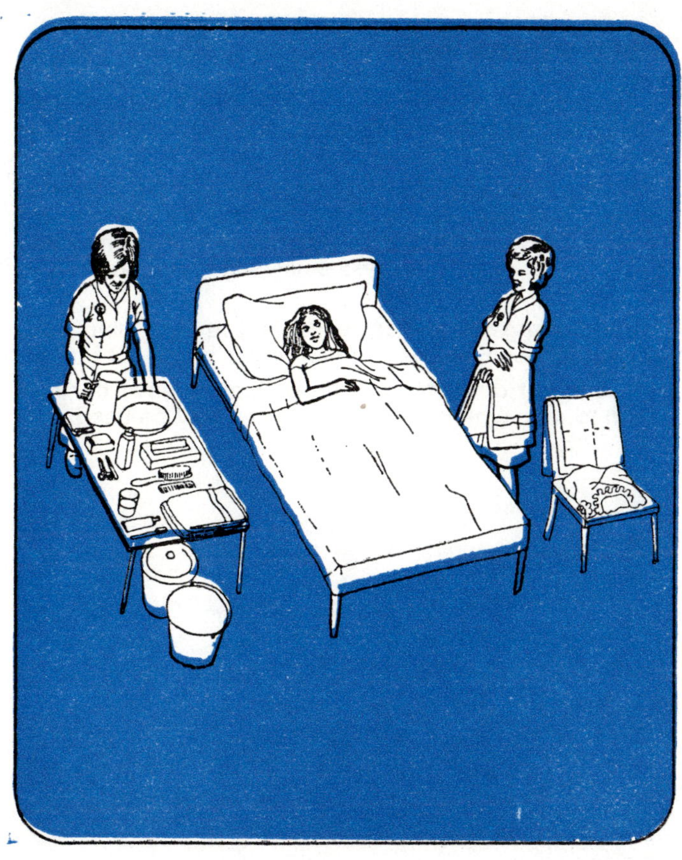

Method

See that the room is warm and the window closed.

Ask the patient if she would like to go to the lavatory (or give a bedpan if necessary).

Remove special equipment in the bed — cradles, footrests, etc.

Strip the bed, covering the patient with one of the large bath towels. Place the other bath towel under her to protect the bed from getting wet.

Help the patient to remove her nightdress or pyjamas leaving her covered with a towel.

Wash, rinse and dry in this order:

> Face, ears, neck, arms, chest and abdomen (tummy), legs, groins (between the legs) and the back.

Uncover each part in turn and cover it again when washed and dried. When washing your patient's hands give her the opportunity to rinse them in the bowl of water.

Cut finger nails and toe nails as necessary. Toe nails should be cut straight across and finger nails rounded to the shape of the top of the finger. Collect the pieces of nail and filings in a paper tissue for disposal.

Treat pressure areas as required (see page 20).

Change the water as soon as it becomes cool or dirty.

Use talcum powder as desired by the patient.

Help the patient to put on clean clothing, to do her hair and to clean her teeth.

Make the bed, removing the large bath towels at the same time.

Make the patient comfortable.

Clean all equipment and put it away tidily.

Open the window as required.

Report any red areas, spots or colour change in the patient's skin which you may have noticed.

A patient who is confined to a chair may be helped to bath in her chair in a similar way.

Care of the mouth

When food is eaten, small particles are left behind after the food is swallowed. These particles decompose and, unless removed, germs flourish and tooth decay may occur. This is especially so if the food eaten is sweet and sugary. The lining of the mouth then becomes inflamed and there is an unpleasant taste. Teeth should be cleaned regularly and, in addition, the mouth rinsed with water after meals to remove any particles. This is especially important if the patient has a high temperature or is eating very little. Under these conditions the mouth becomes furred and unpleasant.

A patient who is ill in bed will require:

- Her toothbrush
- Toothpaste or powder
- A glass of water
- A bowl to spit into
- A towel

Care of the hair

Hair should be brushed and combed into a style which is pleasing to the patient and is easy to manage in bed.

If your patient is ill for a long time ask the doctor or nurse whether it is possible or desirable for your patient to have her hair washed. If permission is given you may find that a local hairdresser is willing to come and do this.

If a hairdresser is not available you may help your patient to wash and set her hair or you may do it for her.

If it is not desirable for the patient to have her hair washed, ask whether a dry shampoo may be used.

To wash the hair of a patient who is not allowed out of bed

(*For Proficiency Certificate*)

Requirements

Waterproof or plastic sheeting to protect the bed
A bowl of hot water
A jug of water for rinsing
A bucket for used water
The shampoo
Towels
A waterproof shoulder cape if available
A small towel for patient's eyes
A hand hair drier if available
The patient's brush and comb.

Method

Explain to your patient how you are going to wash her hair.

Protect the bed with waterproof sheeting and put the shoulder cape round the patient.

Place the bowl on the bedtable in front of your patient, or on the mattress behind her. Wash the hair thoroughly and rinse well. Partly dry the hair using a towel or hair dryer. Set the hair as desired. Completely dry the hair.

Leave the patient comfortable.

Clear away equipment.

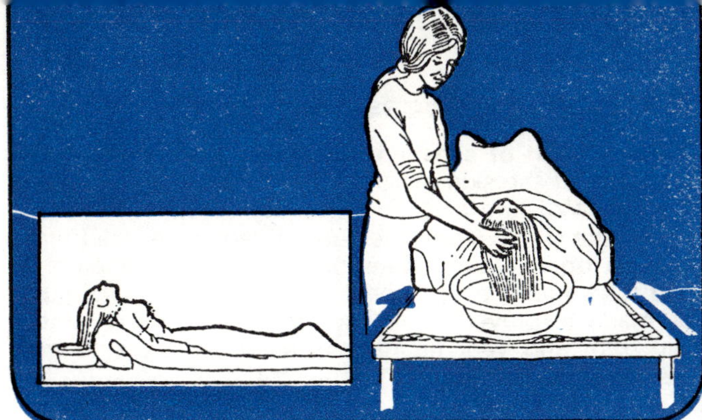

To treat infested hair

(*For Proficiency Certificate*)

A person's hair may be infested with lice. These lay eggs on the hair and reproduce very quickly. To kill the lice, wash the hair with a special shampoo. Alternatively a special cream may be used. Rub this into the hair and leave for 24 hours. Wash the hair. Comb the hair with a fine tooth comb to remove dead lice and nits (eggs). When treating an infested head, your own hair must be protected by keeping it tied back or well covered, so that it cannot come into contact with the hair of the patient. Put brushes and combs into disinfectant. Care must be taken that lice do not spread to other people.

Note: Some of the special creams and shampoos are inflammable and they must be kept away from flames and lighted cigarettes.

Care of the pressure areas

The weight of a patient's body causes pressure on the parts of the skin in contact with the bed and bedclothes. Moisture and friction cause soreness in these areas; the skin becomes red and if neglected will break into an open wound. Pressure sores are very painful and take a long time to heal, so that every effort must be made to prevent their occurrence. Elderly patients, very thin and very fat people are most liable to get pressure sores.

To prevent sores

Change the position of your patient frequently (every 2 hours if necessary).

Keep the skin clean and dry. Pressure areas should be washed and well dried. Apply talcum powder. Use a water silicone, barrier cream or zinc and castor oil if the skin is likely to get wet.

Make the bed well pulling the bottom sheet taut.

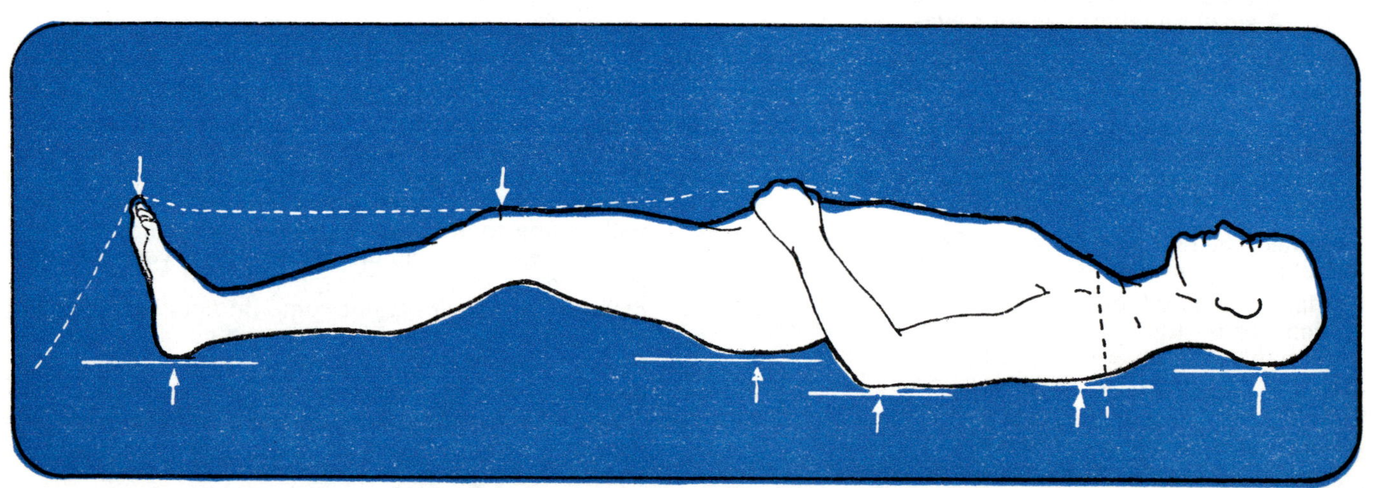

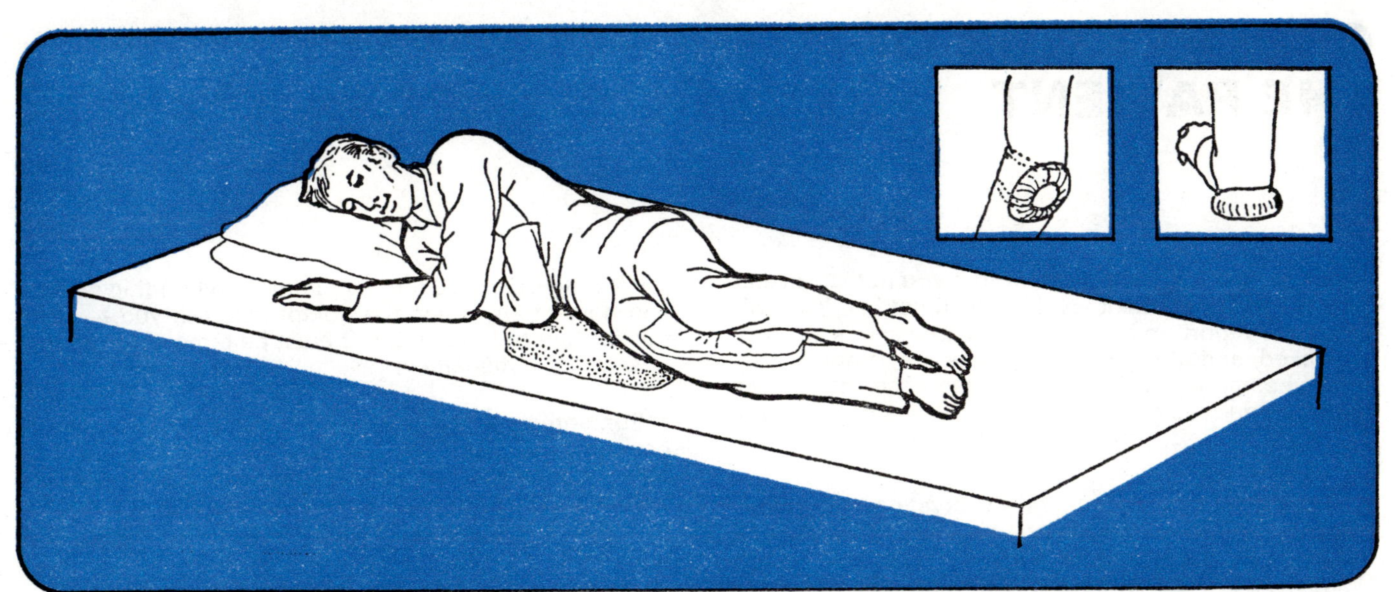

Remove creases and crumbs.

Straighten the clothing under your patient.

Use pillows, pads or rings to relieve pressure.

Natural sheepskin or special wool fleece may be used for the patient to lie on. It is good for this purpose because it contains lanoline which lubricates the skin, is resilient, absorbs moisture, reduces friction, does not wrinkle and is washable.

Special mattresses, some inflatable or electrically operated, are sometimes recommended.

Pressure sores are less likely to occur if your patient eats a well-balanced diet.

OBSERVATION OF THE PATIENT

With experience, you will find that you notice several facts about your patient just by looking at her. You will be able to report on her colour, whether she is anxious or relaxed, and also, by her expression and position in bed, whether she has pain. All these observations are important and the reporting of them will help the doctor and nurse in their work.

In addition to such general observations you must learn to report certain facts, such as the patient's temperature, pulse and respiration rates, how much sleep she has had, whether she has enjoyed her food, how much she has had to drink, whether she has had pain or whether the medicine or pills helped her.

You should also notice if she has a cough and whether anything is coughed up, in which case paper handkerchiefs should be used and then burnt. Sometimes the doctor or nurse may ask you to save such material for them to see on their next visit. Special waxed cartons are available for this purpose.

If a patient is sick, you should note when this occurs and how often. Again the doctor may ask you to save this for him to look at, but it must be removed from the sick-room immediately.

Sometimes when you are helping to care for a patient the doctor may ask whether she has had her bowels open and is passing urine. All these observations are very important, sometimes helping the doctor to make a diagnosis or to prescribe or change the treatment.

You will notice, too, that as the patient begins to get better, her voice gets stronger, she enjoys her food more and she begins to take an interest in what is going on. Your patient will feel much happier then, and you will know how rewarding good nursing can be.

Clinical observations

The rise and fall in temperature, pulse and respiration rates may show progression or regression of the illness or the onset of complications.

1. The temperature

A clinical thermometer is used to take the temperature of a patient. The normal body temperature is said to be 36°-37°C (97°-99°F) but the temperature varies in different parts of the body. The oral temperature is usually 37°C, and the skin temperature, which is usually taken in the axilla, is approximately 0.5°C lower in a healthy person. From this you will see why the same site should be used for the thermometer when taking your patient's temperature over a period of time.

Hypothermia is a very serious condition where the body temperature falls below normal due to shock or exposure to cold. Old people and young babies are particularly prone to this condition.

Pyrexia is the term applied to any rise of body temperature and is usually due to infection.

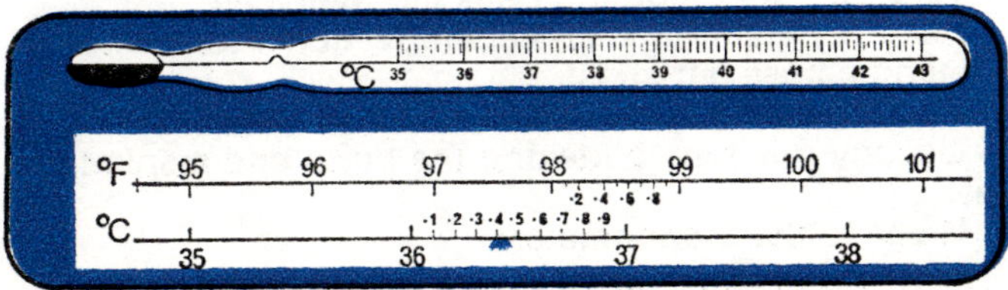

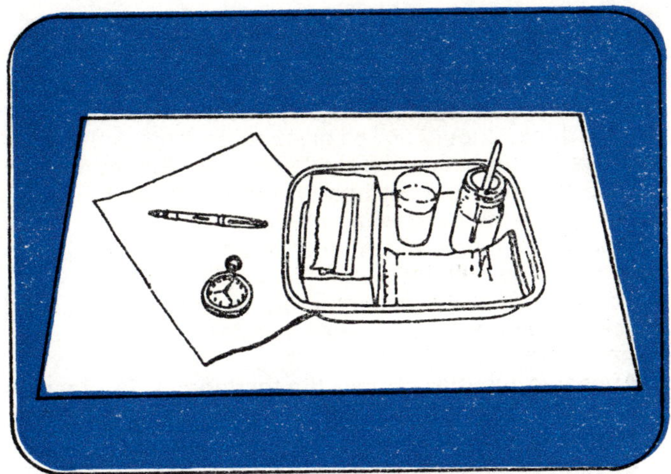

To take a patient's temperature

Requirements on a tray

Clinical thermometer in antiseptic
Cold water in a jar, e.g., paste pot
Cotton wool (or paper handkerchief)
Paper bag for used swabs
Clock or watch with a second hand
Pencil or pen
Paper or temperature chart

The temperature may be taken in the mouth or under the arm (in the axilla).

Method i — By Mouth

Before taking the temperature, pulse and respiration rates, the patient should be lying or sitting quietly. Hot or cold drinks should not be given to patients within 10 minutes before taking the temperature in the mouth.

Take the thermometer from the antiseptic and rinse it in the cold water. Dry with wool or a tissue.

Shake the thermometer until the mercury has gone down into the bulb below the 35°C (95°F) mark.

Place it under the patient's tongue. Ask the patient to close her mouth, but not her teeth, around the thermometer.

After two minutes remove the thermometer and read the level of mercury. This indicates the patient's temperature. Write this down.

Check the temperature recorded on the thermometer before shaking down the mercury with a flick of your wrist.

Rinse the thermometer in cold water and return it to the antiseptic solution.

Remember you must never register any surprise or alarm however high the recorded temperature may be.

Always report an abnormal temperature.

This method cannot be used for any patient who is irresponsible, whether because of age or illness. Neither should it be used for a patient with a mouth injury or one who cannot breathe through her nose.

If any of these conditions exist the skin temperature must be taken.

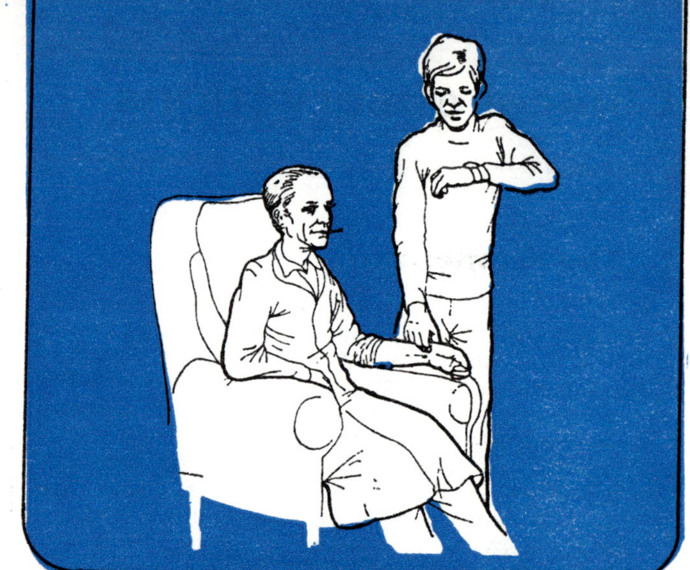

Method ii — in the Axilla

See that your patient is sitting or lying down.

Insert the thermometer under her arm, making sure that the bulb is in contact with folds of skin.

Take care that clothing does not intervene.

Ask the patient to keep her elbow at her side and her forearm across her chest.

Leave the thermometer there for two minutes.

Occupy this time by taking the pulse and respiration rates.

Remove the thermometer.

Proceed as described above.

2. The pulse rate

The pulse is the wave of dilation in an artery caused by contraction of the heart as it pumps blood round the body.

The pulse can be felt wherever an artery crosses a bone near the skin surface.

The radial pulse at the wrist is the one usually taken because it is at a site convenient to patient and nurse.

The average adult rate is 72 beats per minute. In a baby the pulse beats 120-140 times per minute, falling to approximately 80 beats per minute by the age of 12 years.

Remember that the pulse rate increases not only because of some diseases but also after exercise, during fever and in emotional states such as fear.

To count and record the pulse rate

Requirements

A watch with a second hand
Pencil or pen
Paper or temperature chart.

See that your patient is at rest, either sitting or lying down. Put the tips of your first three fingers along the line of the radial artery, just above the creases in the inner aspect of the wrist, and your thumb behind it.

Hold your watch in your free hand and count the rate for one minute. Record the rate.

3. The respiration rate

One respiration consists of breathing in and breathing out.

A newborn baby breathes 30-50 times a minute. This decreases as she get older and the adult rate is 16-20 times a minute.

To count and record the respiration rate

Requirements

A watch with a second hand
Pen or pencil
Paper or temperature chart.

Count your patient's respiration rate for one minute immediately after counting the pulse rate, whilst you are still holding her wrist.

This is so she is not made aware that you are counting her breathing. (It is very difficult not to change one's respiration rate when one knows it is being counted.)

Record this rate.

To use temperature charts

(For Proficiency Certificate)

The temperature, pulse and respiration rates may be taken 4-hourly, if abnormal, otherwise twice a day, at night and in the morning.

These observations should be recorded graphically on special charts, by making a spot in ink at the appropriate level and in the column that indicates the time and date.

The dots on the chart are joined by lines. A tidy chart not only indicates a pride in your work but is much easier for the doctor or nurse to read.

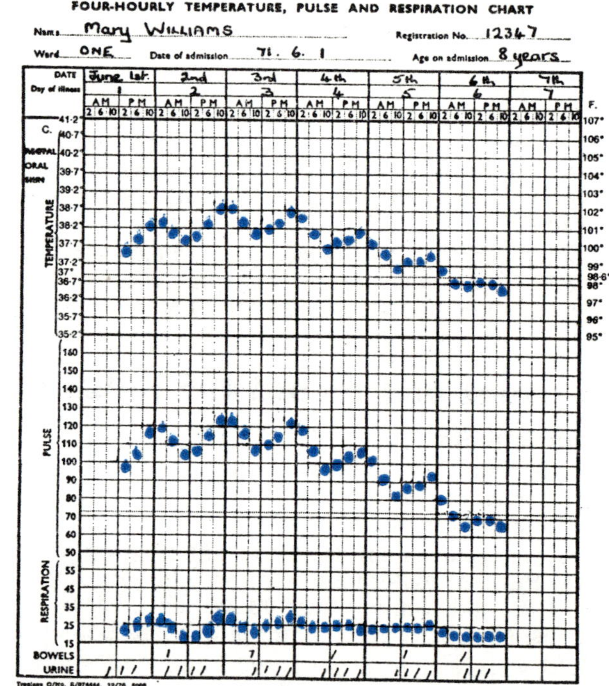

ATTENDING TO THE NEEDS OF THE PATIENT

Vomiting

As well as noting when and how often your patient is sick, it is important to help her whilst she is being sick and to make her comfortable after she has been sick.

To help a patient who feels sick or who has vomited

A patient who feels sick is often frightened and needs to be reassured. See that a bowl and towel are near at hand.

Encourage the patient to breathe deeply. If she is sick support her head and hold the bowl for her.

Remove the vomit from the sick-room immediately.

Wash and dry the bowl and return it to the patient.

After a patient has been sick, wash her face and give her a mouth wash.

If necessary change her clothes and bedding.

Leave her comfortable and warm.

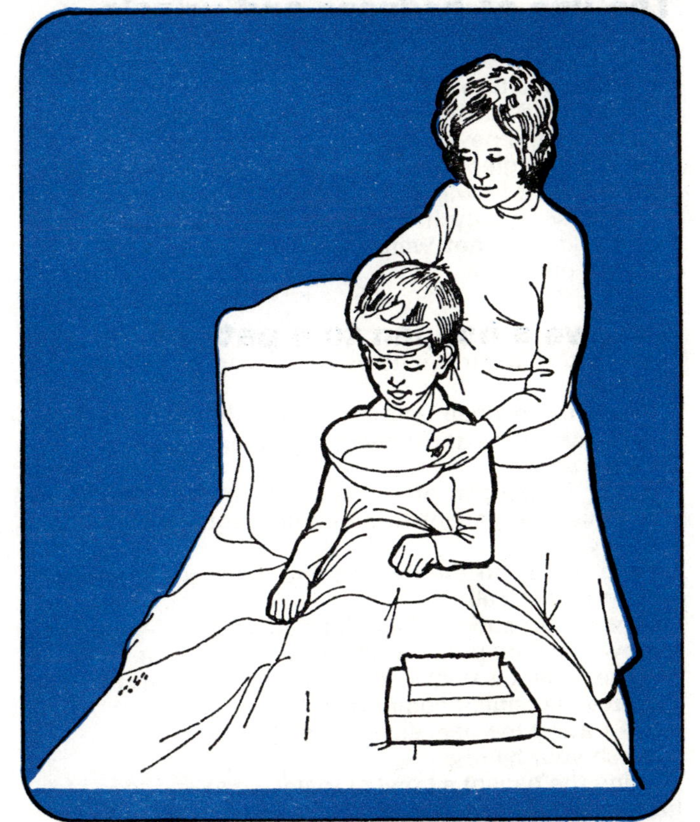

The use of bedpans and urinals

When your patient is unable to get out of bed to go to the lavatory or to use a commode in her room, you may be asked to bring her a bedpan.

This should be kept in the lavatory or bathroom when not in use and never in the patient's room.

Before bringing it to the patient you should make certain that it is warm and dry.

After use, empty it in the lavatory, rinse with cold water and then hot water, using a mop kept for that purpose only.

To give a bedpan to a patient

Close the larger windows and put a screen across the door.

Warm the bedpan with hot water, dry it well, cover it and take it to the patient together with a roll of lavatory paper.

Place the bedpan on a chair, loosen the bedclothes and assist the patient to move her nightgown out of the way.

Help her on to the bedpan and leave the room but remain within call.

When the patient has finished with it, carefully remove the pan, put it on the floor and cover it.

If the patient is unable to clean herself, do this for her.

Leave the patient comfortable.

Take away the pan, empty and clean it.

Wash your hands.

Bring the patient a bowl of water, soap and towel for her to wash her hands.

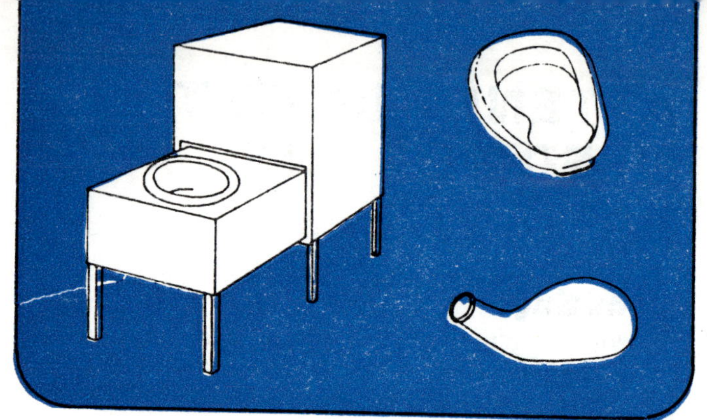

Remove the screen and open the window.

A urinal (a bottle) made of glass or plastic is used by a boy when he passes water. This should be brought to him with a cover, and emptied immediately after use. (A wide-mouthed jar can be used instead of a urinal.)

Again wash your hands and give a bowl of water, soap and towel to the patient to wash his hands.

Incontinence is the term used when someone is unable to control the passing of water or faeces. For example, some handicapped children are incontinent of urine and may have to wear special appliances because of this. Others may use incontinence pads which are disposable pads of wool and other absorbent materials.

Because the skin may get wet and sore, great attention has to be given to keeping it protected, clean and healthy.

ROUTINE OF THE PATIENT'S DAY

The daily routine will depend on the condition of the patient, the patient's wishes and also when help is available.

Anticipate your patient's needs and see that anything she may want, such as books, newspapers, writing materials, spectacles, radio, handkerchiefs, drinks (if allowed) are nearby.

Throughout the day, change the position of the patient frequently. Give medicines and carry out treatments as requested by the doctor or nurse.

See that your patient is able to wash her hands before meals and after using a bedpan.

Your patient may need help with peeling fruit (if allowed). See that she has a plate and knife for this.

See that her letters are delivered or posted promptly.

Remember too that most patients like to talk, so give her an opportunity to do this. Never appear to be so busy that you have no time to listen or to explain.

When helping to look after a sick child, set time aside to play with or read to her. Help her with modelling, drawing or any hobby in which she is interested.

At night time make your patient comfortable and see that she has everything she may need, i.e., a drink and a clock. See that she is able to reach the light and radio switch and a bell should she require help.

THE PATIENT'S DIET

The human body is like a machine — it needs fuel and water to keep it working. The food we eat is fuel for the body. It is broken down in the body to simple substances which are dissolved in water and can be used by the cells to keep them alive and make them work.

A person needs the right quantity of the right foods; age, occupation and weather will influence these needs but in all cases a balanced diet is required.

A balanced diet

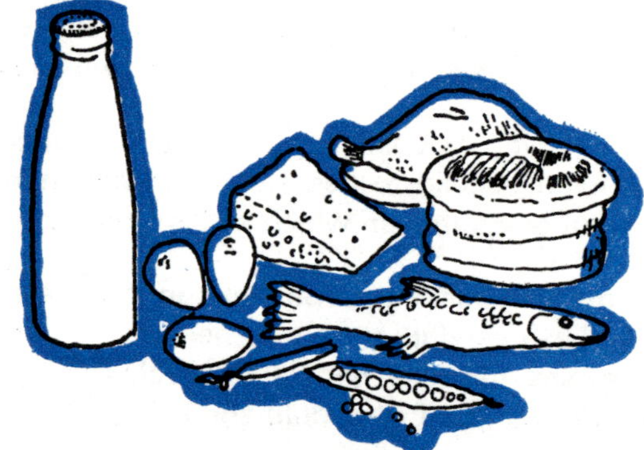

Proteins are essential for growth and repair of the body. The most valuable ones are animal products — lean meat, fish, eggs and cheese. Vegetable sources are peas and beans.

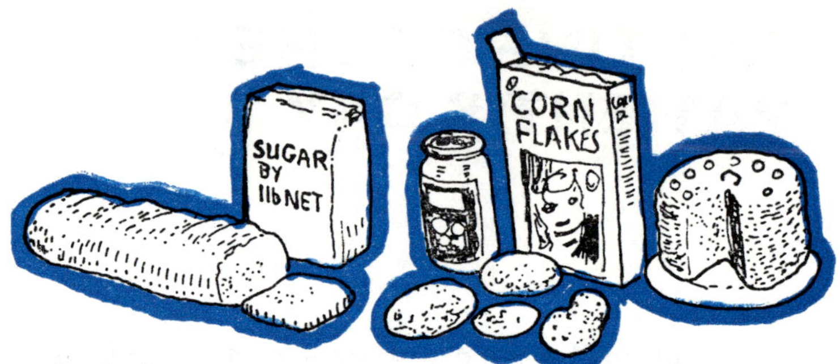

Carbohydrates are fuel foods for immediate energy. They consist of two groups — starches and sugars. The usual sources are rice, bread, potatoes, sweets and fruit sugar.

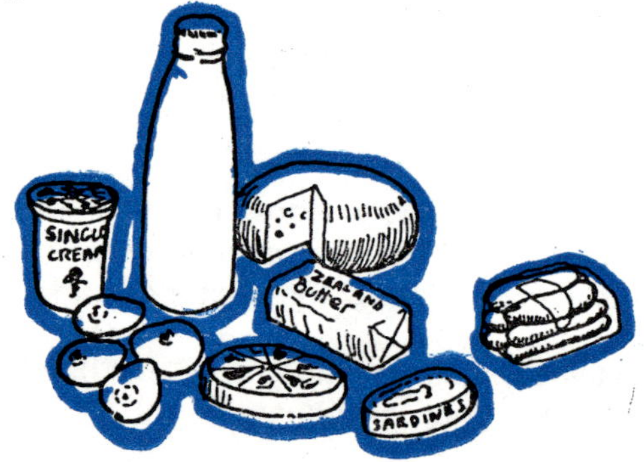

Fats are needed for long-term energy and warmth. They include butter, cream and oils.

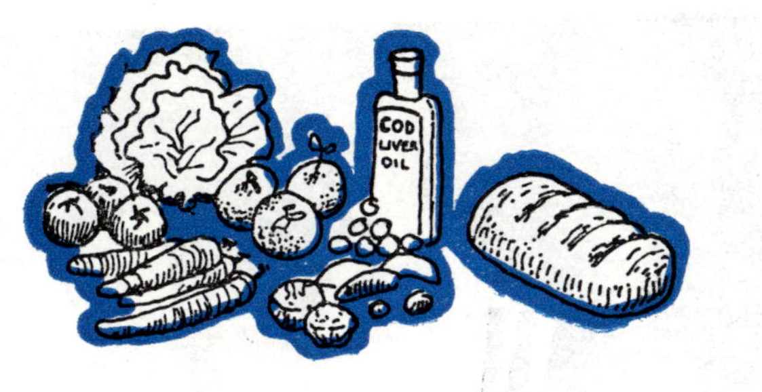

Vitamins are vital for health and growth and include:

- Vitamin **A** found in carrots and yellow fruits (such as apricots), butter, egg yolk, cheese and liver.
- Vitamin **B** found in cereals, bread and liver.
- Vitamin **C** found in some fruits (especially citrus and blackcurrants), green vegetables and potatoes.
- Vitamin **D** found in fats and fish oils. It can also be formed by the action of sunshine on the skin.

Mineral Salts are essential for health and include:

- Sodium chloride (salt)
- Calcium phosphate found in milk and cheese
- Iron found in liver and red meat
- Iodine found in sea fish.

Water is in most foods.

Roughage (indigestible cellulose) is found in vegetables and brown bread.

Special diets

When a person is ill, the cells may not do so much work and the patient does not feel like eating her normal diet. For patients with some illnesses, the doctor will order a special diet.

A fluid diet should include milk, plain or flavoured, fruit drinks and savoury drinks (clear soup or bovril). Milk contains all the essentials of a normal diet. An adult should have a minimum of 3 litres (5 pints) of fluid a day. A cup usually holds 140 ml (5 ounces). A patient with a high temperature needs an increased amount of fluid because she loses fluid by sweating.

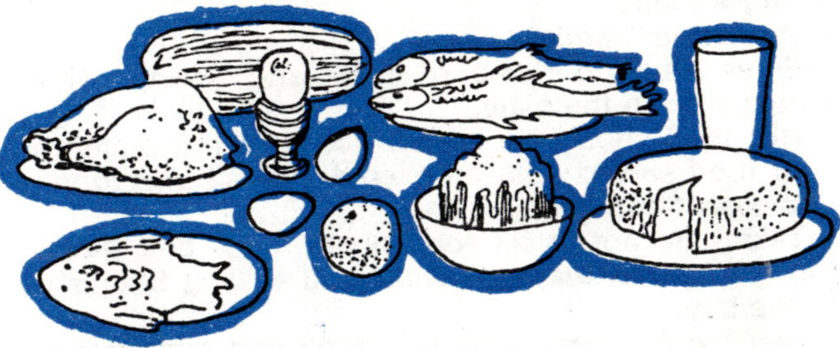

A light diet consists of easily digested foods given in small quantities. It may include milk, eggs, white meat and fish, jelly, custard, ice cream, sponge cake and puréed fruit and vegetables. Fried foods must not be given.

For other diets the doctor usually gives the patient a special diet sheet listing the foods she may have.

To serve meals

Always ascertain what food your patient may eat.

Set the tray with china and cutlery which must be sparkling clean; chipped or cracked china should not be used. A clean table napkin must be provided.

Butter, jam or marmalade may be served in small paste pots to conserve space on the tray.

Place salt, pepper and mustard, if appropriate, in one corner of the tray.

Serve bread or toast on the side plate.

Give a fresh glass of water at lunch and supper times.

See that your patient is in a comfortable position for eating a meal.

Wash your hands.

Serve small portions of food and arrange them attractively on the plate.

Hot food should be served hot on a hot plate and cold food served cold on a cold plate. Tepid food is unpleasant and unappetising.

Take care not to fill soup plates, cups and glasses too full. In this way you will avoid spilling liquids on to the tray.

Serve only one course at a time and remove used plates before serving the next course.

Remember that when one is ill, meal times are very important occasions to which one looks forward. When helping to look after a patient you should do everything possible to ensure that she enjoys her food. Try to think of small ways to make the tray look attractive and the food tempting. For instance, a single flower on the tray

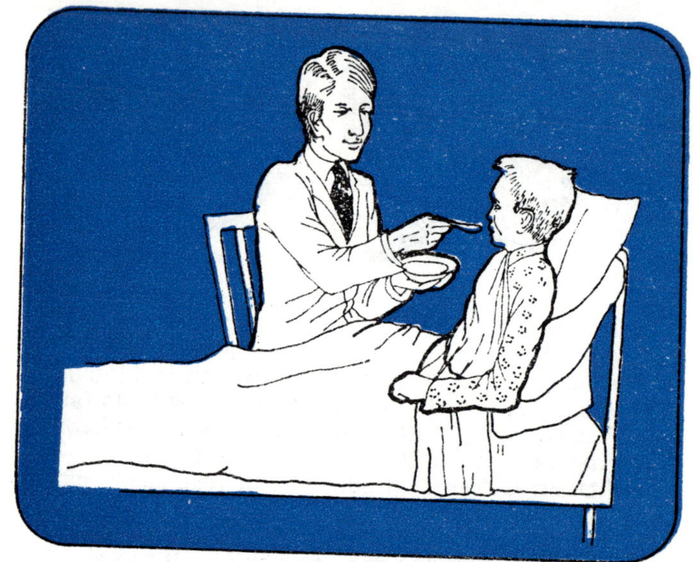

will be appreciated and, if it is available, a small sprig of parsley will make a savoury dish look more appetising, whilst a thin slice of orange or lemon will give a more pleasant appearance to a glass of fruit juice or a jelly.

If the patient is unable to cut up her food herself, this should be done for her quickly so that the food does not become cold.

Sometimes it may be necessary to feed your patient.

To feed a helpless patient

(*For Proficiency Certificate*)

Prepare the patient and the tray as described above.

Bring the tray to the bedside and sit at the patient's side. If you are right handed sit at the patient's right side, and if you are left handed sit at the left hand side of your patient.

Cover the top of the patient's gown and the top of the bed clothes with the table napkin.

Ask the patient if there is anything on the plate which she does not like. Ask whether she likes salt, sugar, etc.

Give small mouthfuls allowing time for her to chew and swallow in between each. To avoid injuring your patient inadvertently with the prongs of a fork, you may use a spoon when feeding her.

When giving fluids, first make sure that they are not too hot. Stand on the patient's right side (if you are right handed) and place your left hand under her head and pillow. Raise her head and give her the drink slowly, holding the cup or feeder with your right hand. Allow time for her to swallow each mouthful.

If your patient cannot drink normally from a cup or feeding cup, it may help to place a straw in the cup or through the spout of the feeder.

For a child lying flat in bed, a special beaker with a lid and a spout may be bought.

As soon as a meal is finished remove the tray and all china and cutlery.

See that your patient is comfortable and has what she needs near at hand.

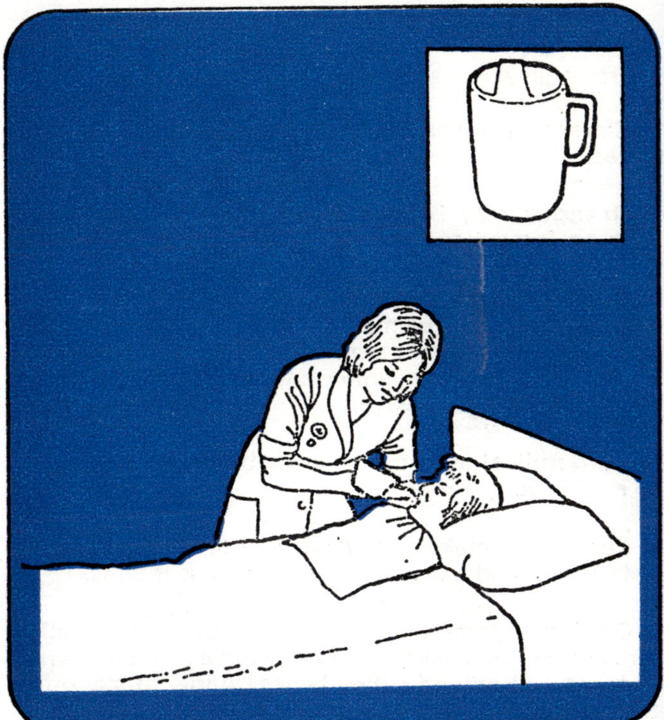

Wash and put away the china and cutlery.
Put away food and containers.

To make drinks

Glasses of squash may be supplemented by fruit juices.

Oranges may be sweetened, strained and served with an ice cube. Sugar may be added as desired or permitted.

Lemonade may be made by simmering the rind of a lemon in half a litre or a pint of water for ten minutes. Add the juice of the lemon and sugar to taste or as permitted. Cool and serve.

Cold milk shakes can be made by adding flavouring to cold milk.

Tea When making tea remember to heat the teapot beforehand and use the water as soon as it boils.

Coffee, if permitted, can be made by pouring half a litre or a pint of boiling water on to three heaped dessert spoonsful of ground coffee beans. Allow to stand for 5 minutes and strain off the coffee.

Hot milk See that milk is hot but do not allow it to boil. Most people find overheated milk unpleasant as fragments of coagulated albumin may appear.

To serve egg dishes

(*Not for examination purposes*)

Eggs are a good standby if your patient does not feel like eating meat or fish.

Boiled eggs Put the eggs into cold water, bring to the boil and cook for 3-4 minutes according to the patient's taste. Use your watch with a second hand if an egg timer is not available.

Poached egg Bring a pan of water to simmering point as you make and butter a slice of toast. Add a few drops of vinegar or lemon juice to the water to keep the egg to a neat shape. Break the egg into a cup and slip it into the pan of hot water. When set, lift it out, drain it well and serve it on the toast.

Scrambled egg Beat 1 or 2 eggs with salt and pepper and a tablespoonful of milk to each egg. Melt 28 grammes (one ounce) of butter in an aluminium saucepan and add the beaten eggs. Stir continuously over a low heat with a wooden spoon until the eggs thicken. Serve on a slice of buttered toast.

Toast Dry toast should be crisp and golden brown. Stand it on edge or in a toast rack to cool. This will prevent toughness.

THE PATIENT'S MEDICINES

Only medicines ordered by the doctor must be given. The patient must always take the full course of medicines or drugs prescribed. You may be asked to give medicines by mouth or by inhalation. Medicines given by injection are given by a nurse or a doctor. Some diabetic patients may give insulin injections to themselves.

In giving medicines to patients you must **check that you:**

Give the	right amount
of the	right medicine
at the	right time
to the	right patient.

Medicines may be given by mouth in liquid or in solid form.

All medicines must be kept in a locked cupboard and put away immediately after use. If a locked cupboard is not available they should be kept on a high shelf well out of the reach of young children. Coloured pills may look like sweets to young children and they may eat them if they are stored within their reach.

Medicines must not be put into bottles or containers other than those in which they are sent from the chemist or doctor. Medicines ordered for one patient should never be given to another even though he has a similar illness.

It is always wise to have a dose of medicine checked by another person before it is given to a patient.

Any medicine left should, with the patient's consent, be dissolved in water and flushed down the lavatory.

To give a liquid medicine by mouth

Read the label on the bottle and check that it is the correct medicine.

Take a suitable measure for the amount ordered (e.g. 5 ml spoon or a medicine glass).

Shake the bottle by putting your first finger on the cork or cap and inverting the bottle several times.

Remove cork or cap holding it in the crook of the little finger throughout.

Hold the bottle with the label facing the palm of the hand (so that the instructions do not become obliterated by drips of the medicine).

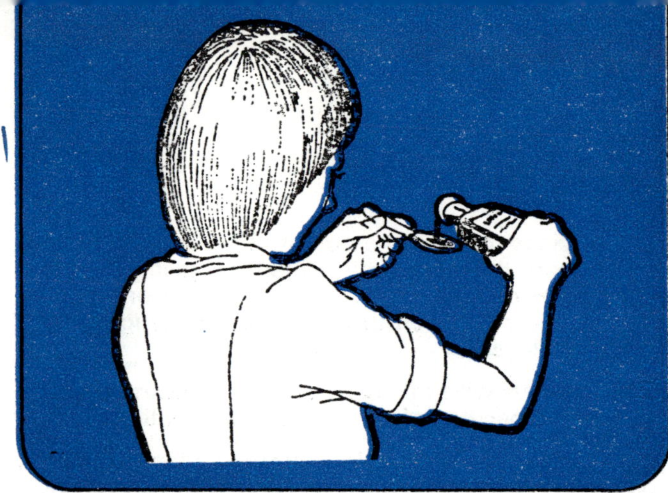

Pour the ordered dose, holding the measure at a suitable level.

Replace the cork or screw cap.

Check the label again.

Take the medicine to the patient and watch her drink it.

Give the patient a sweet or a drink if the medicine is unpleasant to taste.

Wipe the bottle and put it in a safe place out of reach of children.

Wash the measure and put it away.

To give a medicine in solid form

Tablets

Check the bottle contents by reading the label.

Put the required number of tablets into a teaspoon on a saucer.

Check the instructions again.

Take the tablets to the patient immediately and watch her swallow them.

Give her a drink of water.

For children, the tablets may be crushed between two metal teaspoons and the powder mixed with jam or honey.

Capsules or pills (sugar coated) should not be broken but swallowed whole.

Granules are usually chocolate flavoured and may be eaten from a spoon with cereals.

Powders can be mixed in jam or dissolved in water.

To give medicine by inhalation

(*for Proficiency Certificate*)

Sometimes patients are given steam inhalants to relieve the early stages of head colds, sore throats or inflamed air passages (bronchitis). In this way vapour from substances such as Friar's balsam, menthol or pine are breathed in.

For giving inhalations a capsule or a container such as a jug or a Nelson's inhaler is used.

To give an inhalant from a capsule

Cut the capsule with scissors and pour the contents on to several paper handkerchiefs. Hold the handkerchiefs under the patient's nose and tell her to breathe in deeply.

To give a steam inhalant using a jug

Requirements

A litre (or 2 pint) jug
Hot water bottle cover
Flat-bottomed bowl
Measure (e.g. 5 ml spoon kept for the purpose)
Boiling water
The inhalant
Small hand towel.

Method

Sit your patient up to a table and if she is in bed, support her well by pillows.

Place the hot water bottle cover around the jug and to prevent spilling, stand it in the bowl.

Pour half a litre (or one pint) boiling water into the jug.

Measure the inhalant and add it to the water.

Stand the bowl on the table.

Fold the towel like a headscarf around the top of the jug.

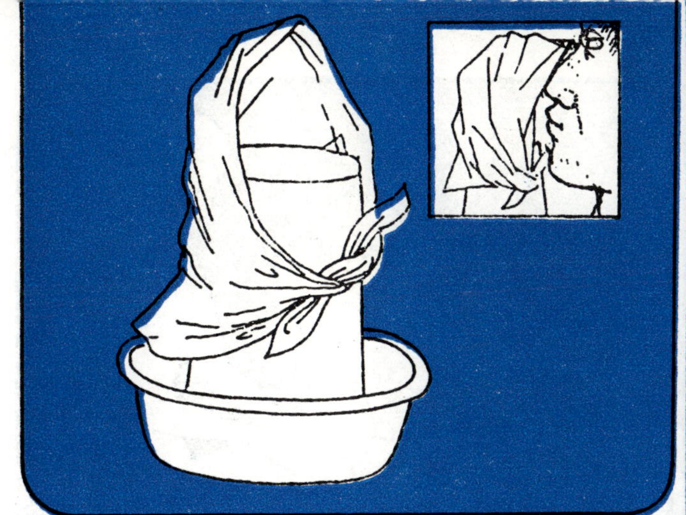

Ask the patient to put her nose and mouth into the opening made by the towel and to breathe deeply for about ten minutes, by which time the water will have cooled. If the patient is unable to lean forward to do this, a dry towel can be placed over her head and the inhaler to form a tent to trap the steam. **This latter method must not be used if menthol is the inhalant as the vapour will irritate the patient's eyes.**

Do not leave the patient alone during the period of inhalation. Hold the bowl and jug if the person being treated is a small child, is very old or cannot for some reason manage it herself.

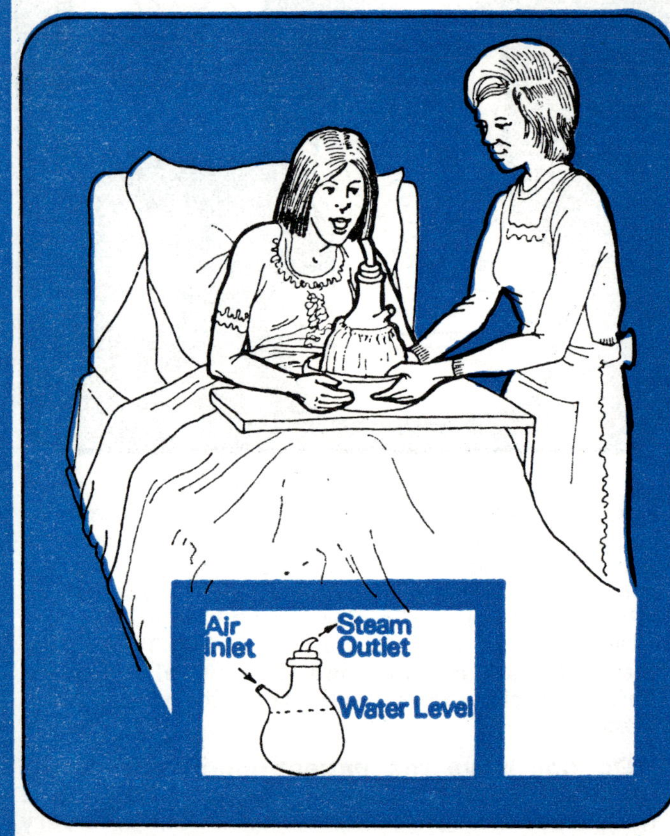

To give a steam inhalant using a Nelson's Inhaler

A Nelson's Inhaler is a special china jug with an air inlet or spout on one side and a steam outlet at the top.

Requirements

Nelson's Inhaler
Hot water bottle cover
Flat bottomed bowl
Measure (e.g. 5 ml spoon kept for the purpose)
Boiling water
The inhalant.

Method

Fill the inhaler with boiling water to the bottom of the air inlet.

Add the inhalant and replace the cork of the mouthpiece in the neck of the inhaler, so that the **spout points in the opposite direction from the air inlet.**

Cover the inhaler at its base and place it in a bowl.

Stand the bowl on a table **making sure that the air inlet faces away from the patient as hot fluid could run out of this and scald her chest.**

Ask the patient to place her lips around the mouthpiece and to breathe in through her mouth and out through her nose.

PREVENTION OF ACCIDENTS IN THE HOME

Preventive nursing is as important as curative nursing, and likewise knowing how to prevent accidents is as important as knowing how to deal with them when they happen.

Some precautions have been mentioned in the previous text. For example, you have already learned that **fires** must always be protected by a fire guard; that **hot water bottles** should be made of rubber, put into a cover and placed outside a blanket in the patient's bed; that **medicines** should be kept in a locked cupboard or put on a very high shelf where a child could not possibly climb; that patients given steam inhalers should never be left alone.

Electric appliances must always be treated with care.

Remember always to switch off before touching any electric appliance. For instance do not pour boiling water from an electric kettle whilst it is still switched on, and do not attempt to remove toast from an electric toaster before switching it off and pulling out the plug.

Read and follow the maker's instructions when using an electric pad or blanket. Always keep it dry, unfolded, and do not stick pins into it.

Electric cords trailing across a room can trip up people, and frayed electric flexes are very dangerous.

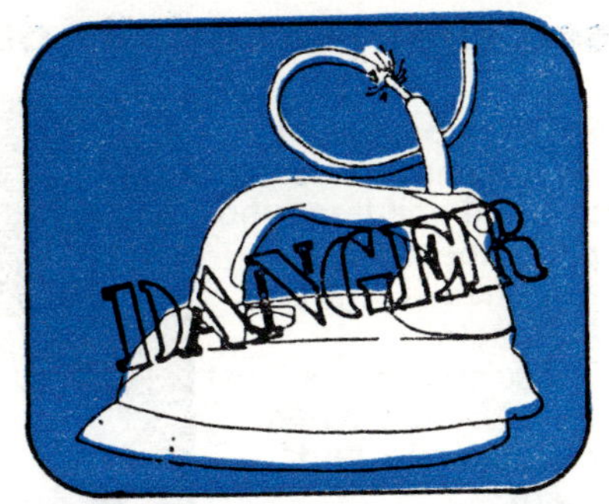

Saucepans and kettles must be kept out of reach and handles kept pointing away from the front of the cooker so they cannot be grabbed by small hands.

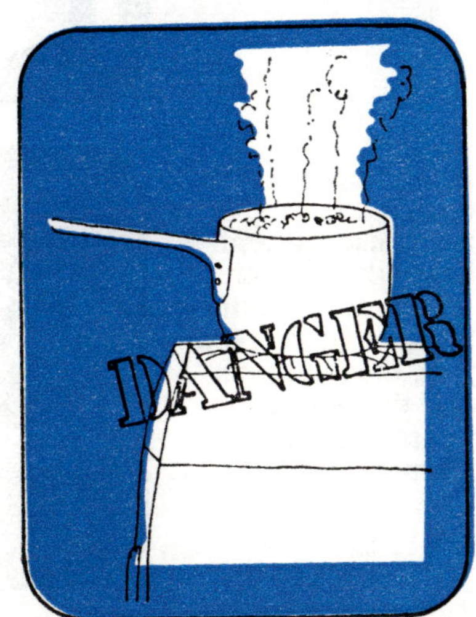

see that potentially dangerous objects are not left lying around

Plastic bags can be the cause of death in small children who place them over their heads and so suffocate.
These containers must never be left where children can find them.

Frayed or loose rugs or carpets, and wet or badly polished floors are dangerous for every-one and especially so for old people and children.

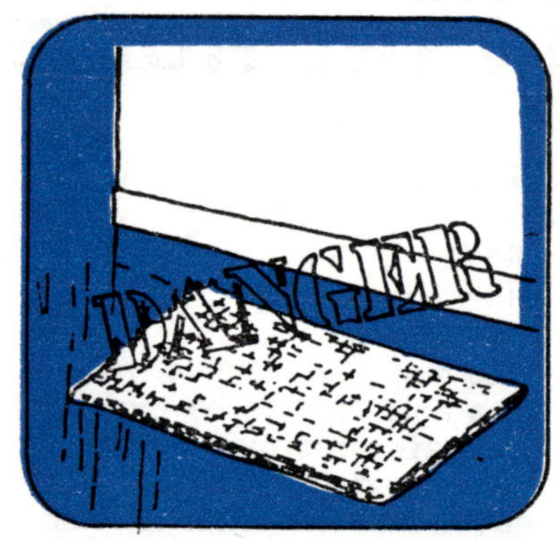

Sharp objects — scissors, knives, etc., must also be kept beyond the reach of young children. If stepped on by bare feet, drawing pins and tin tacks can cause unpleasant injuries.

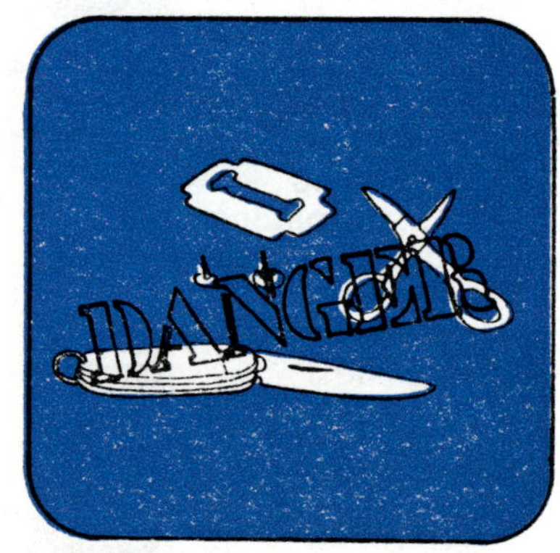

Hot fluids are easily pulled down on top of small children if they are left on a table from which the cloth is dangling.

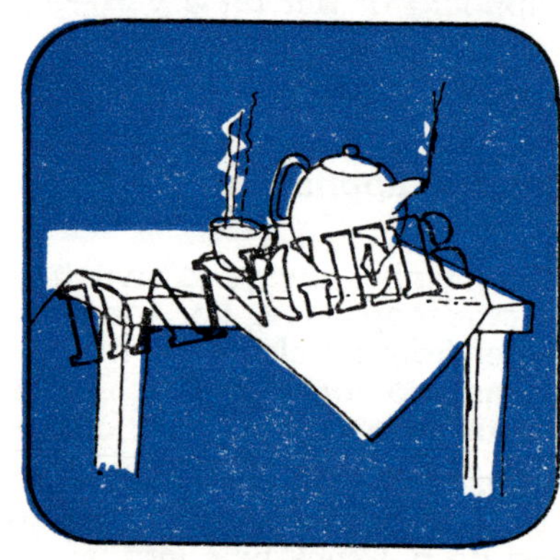

Flames of any kind are another potential danger

Never dry wet towels or clothes in front of a fire — electric or coal — and keep papers and magazines away from that side of the room.

If your patient smokes in bed, see that she has an ashtray and ensure that she does not go to sleep whilst smoking. Flame resisting materials for nightclothes are an added safeguard.

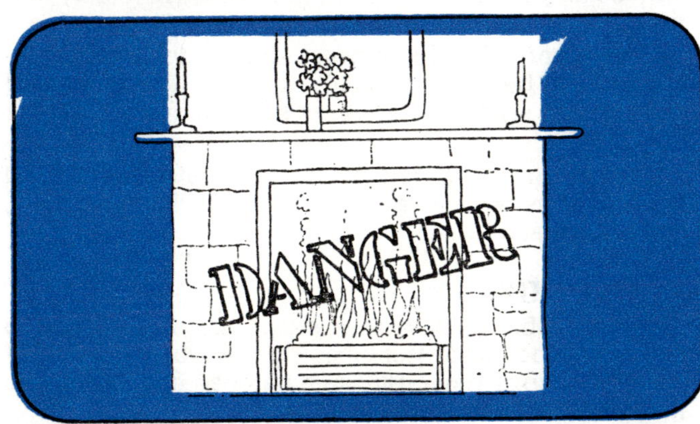

Young children, because they are inquisitive and have not yet learned what is dangerous, are particularly prone to accidents.

In addition to taking care that potentially dangerous objects are not left about, make sure that windows are kept shut at the bottom or blocked so that they can

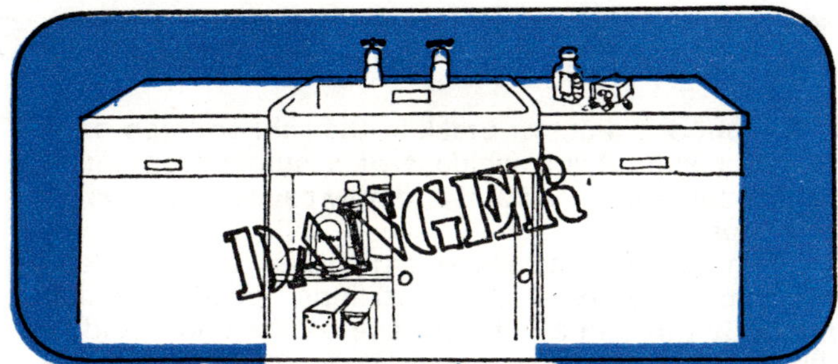

only be opened a short way. Even if you think the window is too high for a toddler to reach, remember small children love climbing, and one might drag a chair to the window and climb up on it to bring him into line with the open window.

Remember also that it is not only medicines which can be eaten or drunk with disastrous results to children. Cleaning fluids and bleaches are just as dangerous and must be kept out of their reach.

When using perambulators or wheelchairs, check the brakes and, if they are in doubtful order, ask a colleague to steady the vehicles for you.

The list of accidents that can happen is very, very long. You will inevitably think of some which are not given here. Whatever they are, part of the service you can give is to do everything you can to prevent such things from happening. It is important at all times, but especially so if you are living with very young or very old people.

THE CARE OF WOUNDS

A wound is a cut or break in the skin and can occur as the result of an accident or a surgical operation. Germs can enter a wound and may cause inflammation and sepsis.

Germs are minute living organisms which multiply very rapidly in favourable conditions. When they enter the body through a cut, they live on the body fluids in the heat of the body and multiply rapidly to form sepsis. The white blood cells respond to this infection by going to the site to destroy the germs.

When caring for a wound, doctors and nurses use an aseptic (without sepsis) technique to prevent the entry of germs.

Sterilisation

Sterilisation is the means by which germs are killed to render equipment and dressings sterile.

Equipment is often sterilised by the manufacturer and this is carried out by exposing the instruments, etc., to gamma radiation from a nuclear reactor. The equipment is sealed into a plastic or paper covering and it remains sterile until the seal is broken.

Dressings, foil and plastic containers for lotions are also sterilised in this way and are available in sterile packets.

When pre-sterilised equipment is not available other methods of sterilisation may be used.

Boiling can be used for metal, glass, china and enamelware. Absolutely clean equipment is placed in a clean container (e.g. saucepan) and water is poured over to immerse the equipment completely, making sure there are no air bubbles. The water is boiled and must stay boiling for at least three minutes (preferably ten minutes).

Chemical disinfectants, sold under proprietary names, may be used for plastic equipment and for metal instruments. The manufacturer's instructions must be followed.

Steam under pressure in an autoclave can be used for dressings which are packed in special containers, usually metal drums.

Dressings

It is possible to buy small sterile dressings from the chemist to be used after cleaning the wound. Some of these dressings have adhesive patches and others are incorporated with the bandage.

Packets of sterile cotton wool and gauze for both cleaning and dressing wounds are also available from chemists.

If it is impossible to obtain sterile dressings, make sure that the material (white linen or cotton cloth) used is as clean as possible. Washing and ironing destroy many bacteria.

To treat minor injuries - cuts and scratches

Wash and dry your hands to prevent carrying infection to the wound, and then collect the following:

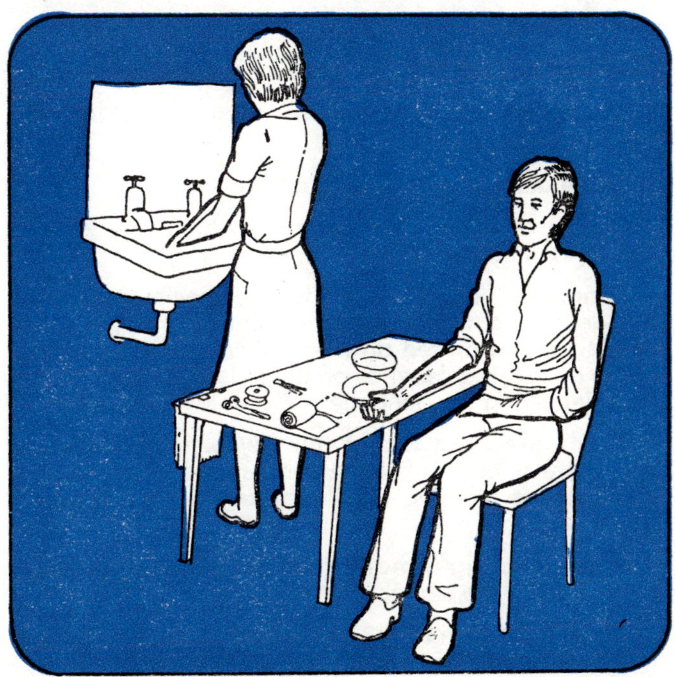

Requirements — on a tray or on a towel on the table.

Wool swabs
Gauze dressing or a clean piece of material
Antiseptic lotion in a bowl
Bandage or plaster
Scissors
Paper bag for soiled swabs.

Method

Tell the patient what you are going to do.

Wash and dry your hands again.

Dip the swabs into the lotion.

Wash very carefully and gently around the wound; always wash away from the wound and do not let water run into it.

After you have used a swab put it into the paper bag; never use a swab more than once.

When the skin is quite clean, cover it with the dressing, taking care not to finger the part of the dressing which covers the wound.

Secure it in place.

If the wound is bleeding, allow it to bleed briefly to wash away any dirt, before bandaging it firmly.

If the wound is septic, the doctor or nurse will tell you what to do.

Soiled dressings should be wrapped in newspaper or paper towels and burnt. If an open fire is not available, the soiled dressings should be wrapped in three thicknesses of paper and put in the refuse bin. In some areas the Local Authority provides a service for the collection and disposal of such material.

BANDAGING

Roller bandages are made of cotton, muslin, flannel, crepe, or special paper.

Widths used: 5 cm (2 in) - for the head
5-7 cm (2-3 in) - for arms and legs

The width of the bandage varies with the size of the patient and the part to be bandaged.

Bandages are used: to keep dressings in position
to provide support
to restrict movement.

Rules for bandaging

Choose the correct bandage and a small safety pin or plaster to fasten.

Make the patient comfortable.

Support the part to be bandaged in the position required.

See that the dressing is in position.

Hold the bandage with the roll uppermost close to the part.

Apply the bandage from below upwards and from inner to outer side of the limb.

Bandage firmly without constricting the part.

Start with one straight turn to fix the bandage.

Each subsequent turn covers two-thirds of the bandage of the previous one.

Finish the bandage with a straight turn and secure the end with a small safety pin (put your fingers between the bandage and the patient to fix the pin so that you do not prick the patient), or a piece of plaster.

Patterns used in roller bandaging

Simple spiral used for a part of the body of uniform size, e.g. the upper arm.

Spica used for a joint, e.g. elbow, knee.

Figure of eight used for parts which vary in size, e.g. forearm, leg or ankle.

Tubular gauze is applied with a special applicator. The gauze is cut to two or three times the length to be bandaged and placed on the applicator. The tightness of the bandaging depends on the twist of the applicator when applying the bandage.

Elasticated net is a stretch net bandage which is also tubular and is stretched over the dressing. No applicator is required (*not necessary for examination purposes*).

A conforming bandage can be used over irregular surfaces, e.g. the ear.

Clear adhesive tape can be used to keep a dressing in place on the ear or eye.

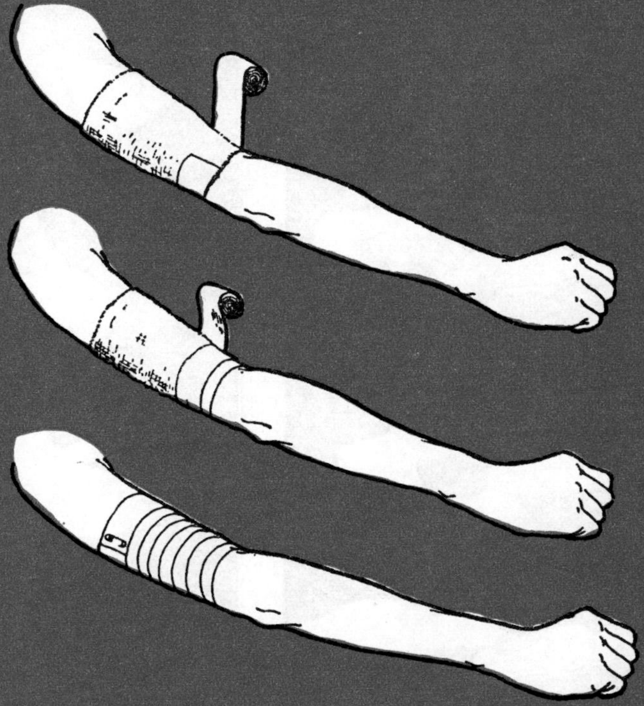

Simple Spiral

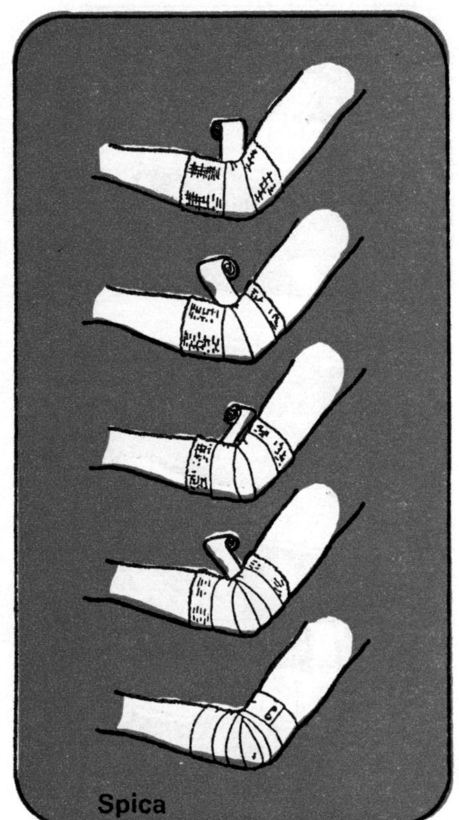

Spica

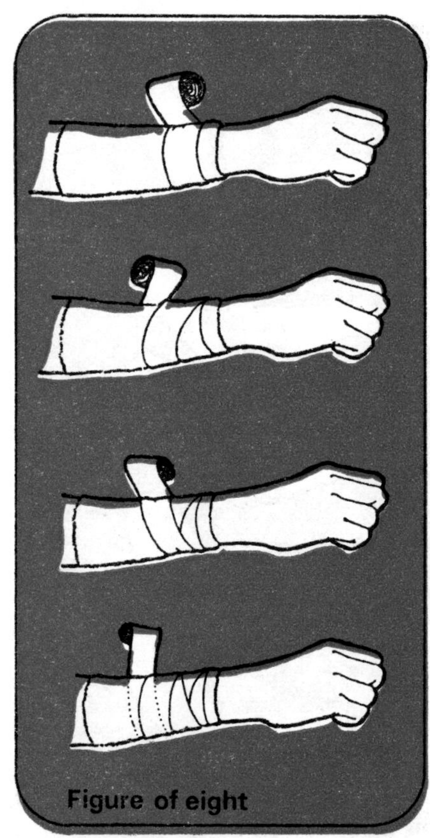

Figure of eight

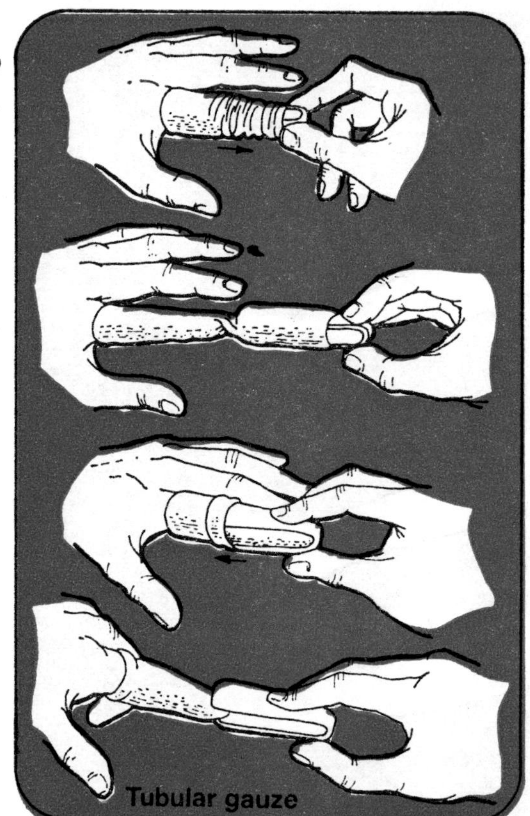

Tubular gauze

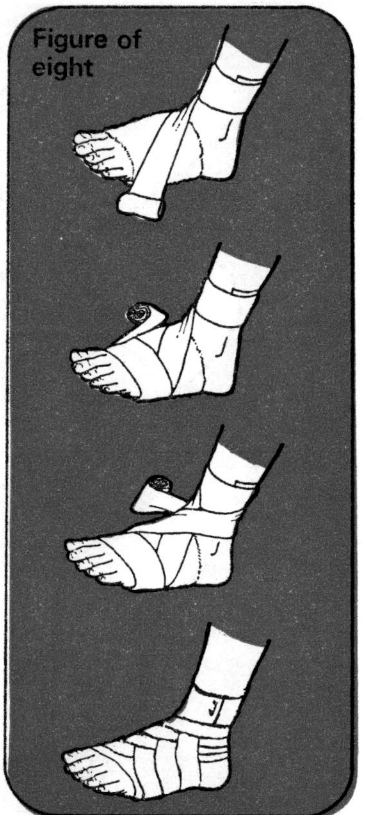

Figure of eight

THE TREATMENT OF INFLAMMATION

Inflammation is the way in which the body responds to infection, injury, heat, cold or chemicals. In infection, germs enter the body as, for example, through an abrasion and cause sepsis as on a septic finger or a boil. Inflammation may be caused by injury, by sunburn or frostbite or by the frequent use of detergents. The part usually becomes swollen, red and hot due to the increased blood supply. This causes pain and the patient has difficulty in using the inflamed part. She may feel ill and have a rise in temperature and pulse rate.

General treatment

Give plenty to drink. (Adults should have at least 3 litres (5 pints) a day.)

Rest — sometimes complete rest in bed is ordered.

Antibiotics to kill germs } ordered by the doctor
Drugs to relieve pain }

Local treatment

This may be by the use of frequent applications of warmth by warm cotton wool, a well covered hot water bottle or Kaolin poultice, or by applications of cold, e.g. cold compress.

A Kaolin poultice is made from a clay paste containing medicated oils which retain heat.

TO APPLY A KAOLIN POULTICE

Requirements

A tin of Kaolin paste
A sauce pan of boiling water
A spatula or metal knife
A piece of old linen of appropriate size
Cotton wool of slightly larger size than the linen
A bandage
A safety pin or adhesive plaster.

PROFICIENCY

PROFICIENCY

Method

Tell the patient what you are going to do.

Remove the lid from the tin of Kaolin.

Place the tin in boiling water so that water comes two-thirds of the way up the tin.

Keep the water heated and from time to time stir the Kaolin with a spatula or knife so that the medicated oil is thoroughly mixed with the clay.

When the Kaolin is hot, spread it on the old linen ½ cm (¼ in) thick. Turn over the edges of the linen.

Take the poultice, cotton wool and bandage to the patient's bedside immediately.

Always test the heat of the poultice on your forearm before applying it to the patient to avoid burning her. Wait for the poultice to cool until you find it comfortably bearable on your forearm.

Place the poultice in position, cover with cotton wool and bandage in place.

Make the patient comfortable.

Clear away all equipment.

Renew the poultice as often as ordered by the doctor or nurse.

TO APPLY A COLD COMPRESS

Requirements

Old linen

Cold or iced water (or eau de Cologne or spirit if the injury is not on the face).

Method

Tell the patient what you are going to do.

Wring out a double fold of the linen in the water or spirit and apply to the injured part.

Renew the compress as soon as it becomes warm.

Remember that spirit must not be applied to areas near the eyes or to the face.

HELPING WITH THE CARE OF INFECTIOUS PATIENTS

Germs are minute living organisms which multiply very rapidly in suitable conditions — warmth, moisture and where there is food. Some germs are useful and act on milk and grape juice to make cheese and wine. Others are harmful and can cause diseases. Germs enter the body via the nose, the mouth or the skin. Germs entering the body may be killed by the white blood cells, by antibodies or by the juices of the body. For example, a germ entering the stomach can be killed by the acid produced in the stomach. Poor general health, lack of food, or lack of sleep prevent the destruction of germs, and dirty conditions encourage their rapid growth.

Infection may be spread by contact with an infected person, by droplets from their coughs and sneezes, by contaminated hands or food, by infected books and toys and by bites from some insects.

Common infectious diseases include influenza, sore throats, chicken pox, measles, mumps, food poisoning and dysentery. (See also Appendix.)

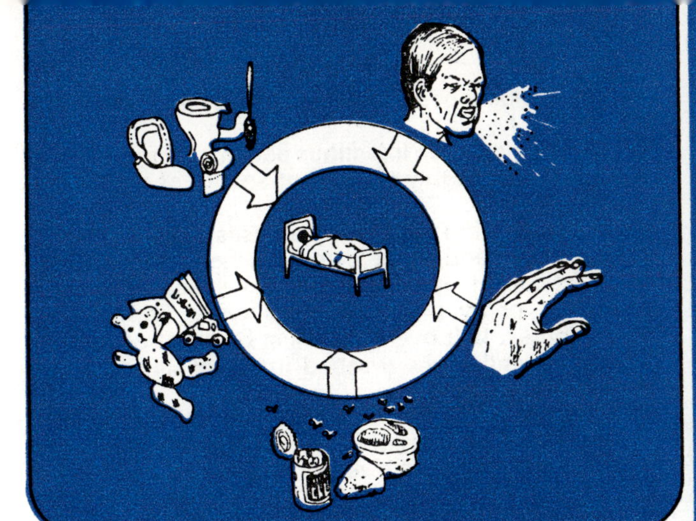

Care of patients suffering from an infectious disease

The patient, where possible, is nursed in a room on her own and visitors are restricted.

Some patients will be admitted to hospital.

The patient should be nursed in bed while her temperature is raised.

The bedroom should be kept clean, well ventilated and free from flies.

A light diet and plenty of fluids should be given. Other treatment will be ordered by the doctor or nurse. A report on the patient's condition should be given to the doctor when he visits.

After attending to an infectious patient you must wash your hands thoroughly to prevent spread of the infection.

Separate drinking and eating utensils should be kept for the patient and, after being washed (separately), may be sterilised by immersion in a sterilising liquid, e.g. Milton, or by placing in cold water and boiling for 10 minutes. Left over food must be burnt or buried.

Bed linen should be washed in hot water and put into the fresh air to dry.

Because of infection, papers and magazines which have been read by the patient should be burnt after use. Library books should be returned to the library in a sealed plastic bag and an explanation given to the Librarian.

Toys given to infectious children should be washable. Inexpensive ones should be burnt after use.

TO PREVENT THE SPREAD OF DROPLET INFECTION — as in colds or sore throats. Paper handkerchiefs should be used by the patient and then placed in a paper bag and burnt.

TO PREVENT THE SPREAD OF INTESTINAL INFECTION (diarrhoea and vomiting)

If the infection is in the faeces it may be necessary to cover the stool with a chemical disinfectant and leave it to stand before disposing of it down the lavatory pan. The bed pan and urinal should be kept only for the patient's use. The lavatory and bath will also need to be disinfected every time they are used.

When the patient is no longer infectious, she should have a bath and put on clean clothing and her hair should be washed. The bed linen should be washed and dried in the air, mattress and pillows put in the fresh air or, in some cases, the Local Authority will take them away to be fumigated before re-use. The furniture and room should be cleaned thoroughly and the window left open for a day.

Prevention of infection by immunity

Immunity is the ability to resist infection. A person who is immune to an infectious disease will not suffer from the disease even when in contact with those particular germs. When a person suffers from an infectious disease, antibodies are formed in the blood to attack the germs. When the patient recovers some of these antibodies remain.

In immunisation the person is given a preparation which will stimulate the production of antibodies and make him immune to that disease.

In the United Kingdom immunisations to the following infections are available to all children: diphtheria, whooping cough, tetanus, smallpox, tuberculosis, measles and poliomyelitis.

Immunisation for diseases like typhoid fever and yellow fever can also be given to people travelling to other countries.

HELPING WITH THE CARE OF SICK CHILDREN

All children need love and security. This is particularly so when they are ill. They may be sick from an infection or they may have had an accident which keeps them in bed. Some children have diseases which make them ill for long periods.

When you are helping to nurse these sick children, all the general nursing care which has been described will need to be carried out as required and in addition a sick child will need someone to talk to or play with, or just for company.

How to keep a child occupied when she is confined to bed

Interesting activities may include playing cards, games like snakes and ladders, building models, sewing, knitting, stamp collecting and jigsaw puzzles. The children's section of many public libraries lends books on paper cutting and toy making.

HUMMING BUTTON

or 1 circle of coloured cardboard

1. Cut a piece of cotton about 2 metres (2 yards) long and double it.
2. Thread it through a button (or cardboard with two holes) which should be at least 3 cm or 1 inch in diameter.
3. Bring the cotton back through the other hole of the button and knot the two ends together.
4. Holding a loop on the forefinger of either hand, twist the button round, then pull on the loops and relax rhythmically and the button will spin round, humming.

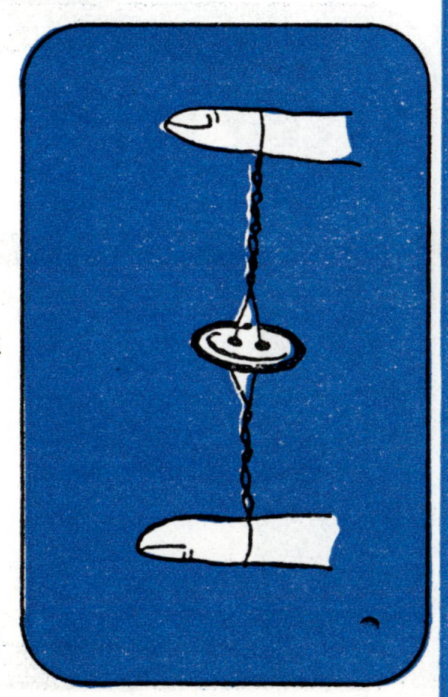

DESIGNING PATTERNS

In coloured cotton on ceiling tiles, cardboard or wood

1. Place pins in tile or cardboard.
2. Tie cotton to one pin.
3. Continue taking cotton round pins to form a pattern.

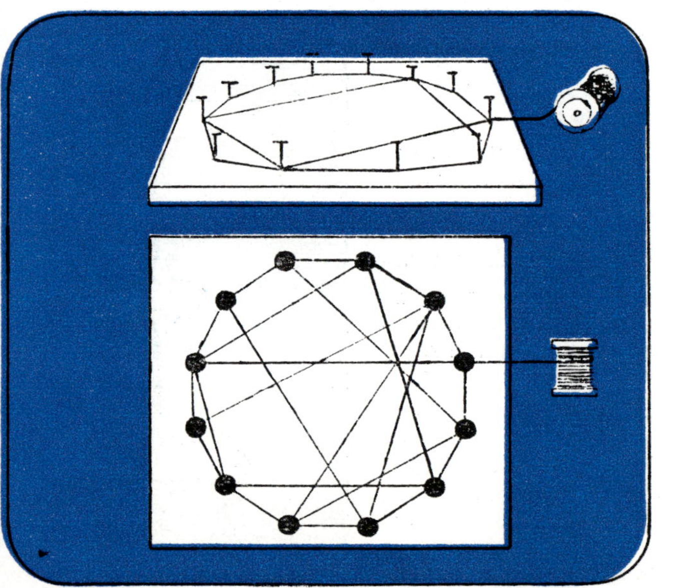

MOBILES

1. Cut out the shape required.
2. Paint and fold top half down.
3. Join by threading cotton through bottom of one shape and top of the next.

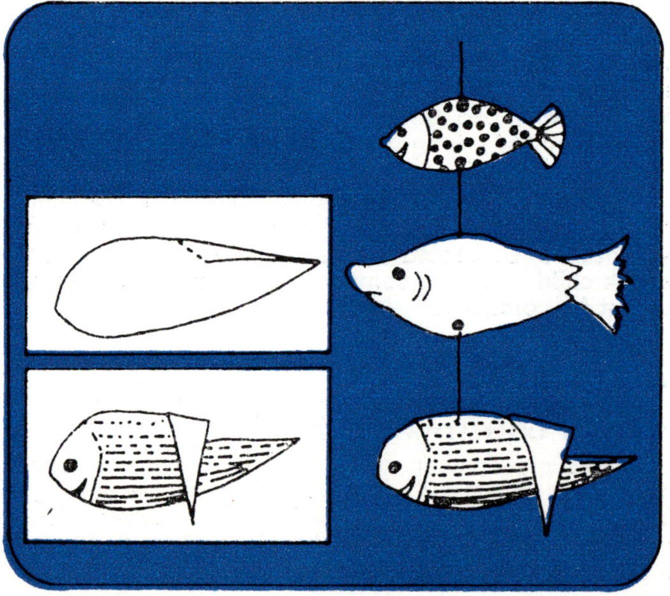

COLLAGES

These can be made of cloth, wool, match sticks, straw, ribbon, paper, seeds and shells. Stick these on a background of cardboard, felt or firm material to make the desired picture.

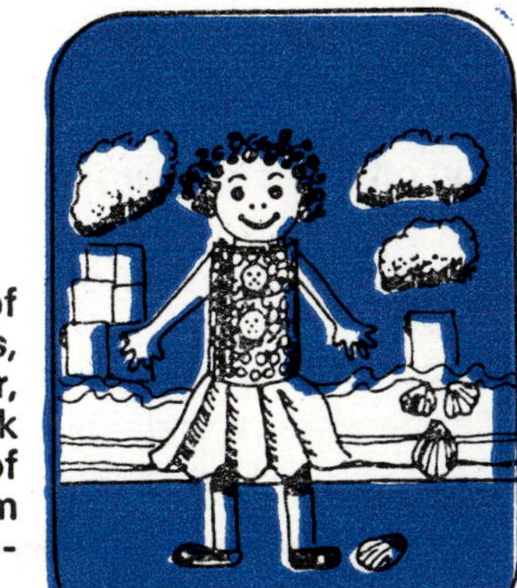

KNITTED BLANKET SQUARES

Different coloured wools can be used in plain knitting. For Red Cross blankets knit squares measuring 15 cm by 15 cm (6 in square) and join together.

GROWING PLANTS

1. Use yoghurt pot or detergent container of plastic, cutting the top off the latter.
2. Fill with soil.
3. Plant seeds or pips, carrot or pineapple tops in containers.

MATCHBOX VILLAGE

Cardboard roof on box
Two matchboxes; cardboard or button wheels

TREES

(i) cut 2 pieces of paper
(ii) slot down centre
(iii) slot one on top of the other
(iv) put trunk of tree into cotton reel.

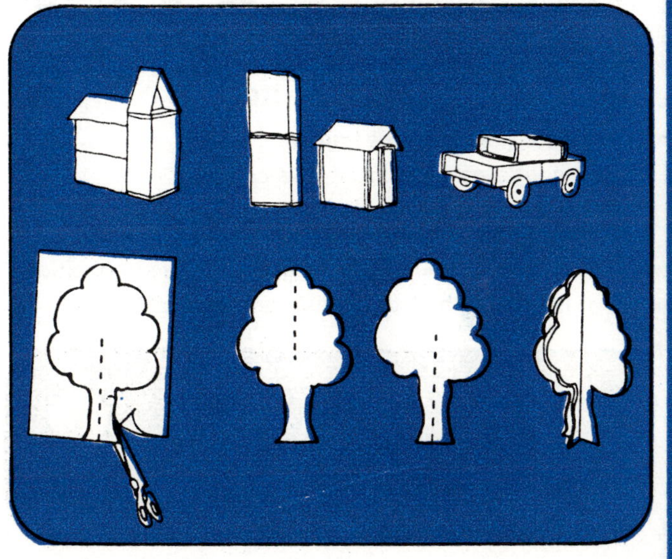

PROFICIENCY

FUN WITH FIGURES

1. Use cylindrical piece of cardboard (such as the core of a toilet roll) and a ball (e.g. table tennis ball).
2. Gum ball to top of cylindrical tube.
3. Paint face and dress.

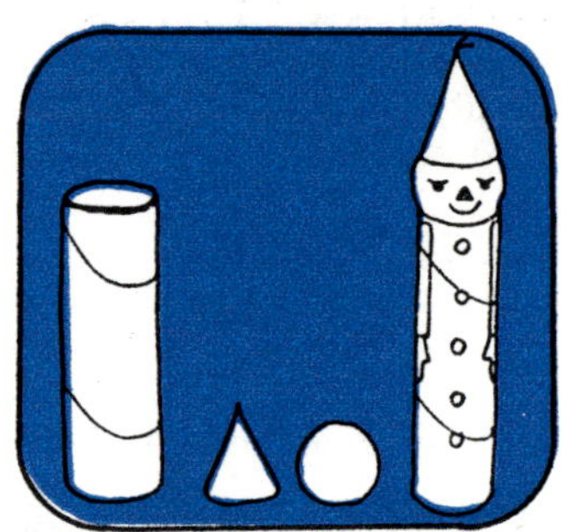

BALANCING BOYS

1. Take two table tennis balls.
2. Cut a little off the top of one ball.
3. Put plasticine in the bottom so that it rocks from side to side.
4. Place second ball on top of first and glue in position.
5. Paint face on ball and dress as required.

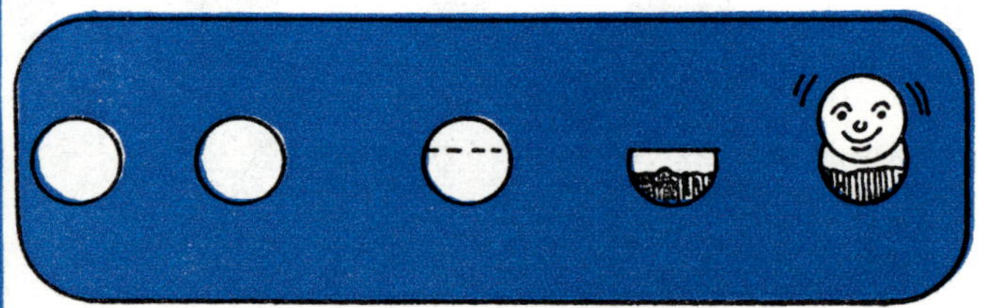

WHIRLIGIG

1. Use a roll of coloured crepe paper, clothes peg, string.
2. Cut off 3-4 cm ($1\frac{1}{2}$ in) of paper and make into roll.
3. Tie string to wire part of clothes peg.
4. Make a loop on other end of string to put finger through.
5. Attach clip to one end of roll of paper.
6. Let paper drop and whirl in the air.
7. After use, roll paper up again.

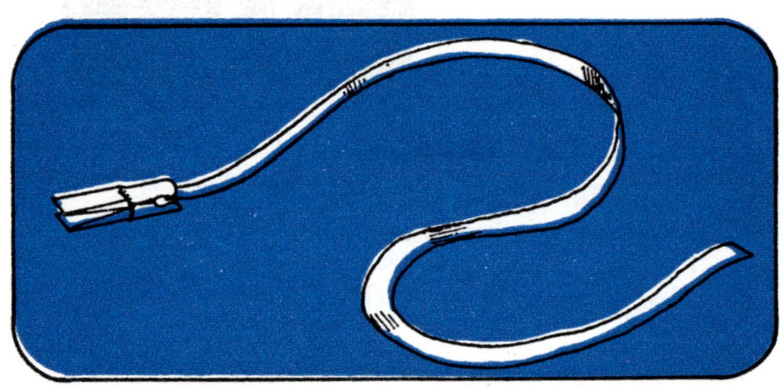

PRECAUTIONS

Do not put toys out of reach so that a child will climb or get out of bed to get a toy.

Do not let a small child use sharp tools such as pointed scissors: plastic ones will cut paper.

CHILDREN'S TELEPHONE

1. Make the telephone out of two tins, approximately 7 or 8 cm (3 in) in diameter.
2. Take the top off each tin and bind the cut edge with adhesive tape.
3. Pierce a small hole in the other end.
4. Cut a piece of string the length of the required distance between the two telephones.
5. Thread the string down through one of the tins and up through the other, knot the ends so that they do not slip back through the holes in the bottom.
6. One person talks into a tin at one end while the other holds the string tight and listens with his ear to the tin at the other end.

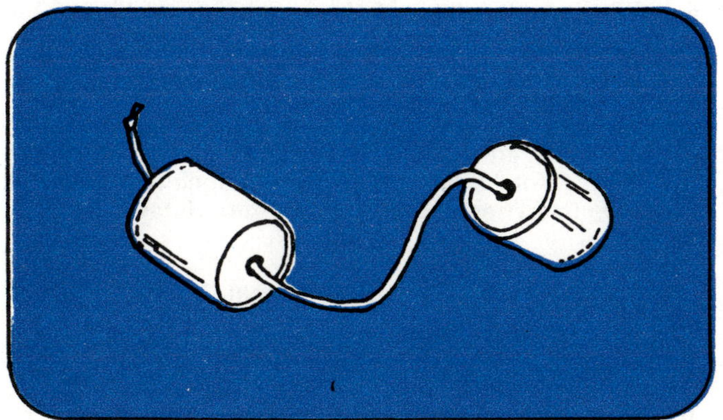

ACORN TOYS

Acorns can be made into small toys, such as human figures, pigs, snakes and prams.

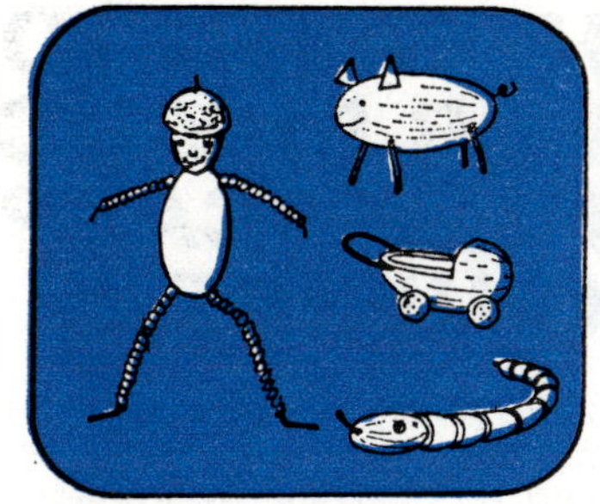

PAPER DRAGON

1. Cut out of stiff paper. 1 metre (or 1 yard).
2. Fold X over Y at right angles.
3. Then fold Y over X and X over Y and so on.
4. Draw on eyes, open out and fix red forked tongue.

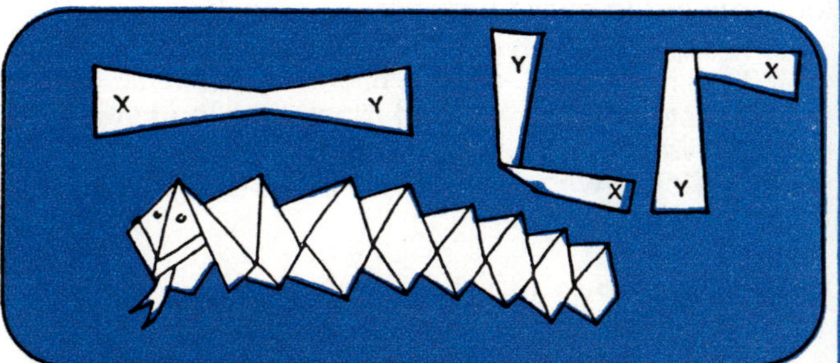

Further suggestions will be found in "Toys and Ideas for Children when ill", a free booklet published by James Galt & Co. Ltd., 30/31 Great Marlborough Street, London, W.1.

PROFICIENCY

HELPING TO CARE FOR PHYSICALLY HANDICAPPED CHILDREN

Physically handicapped children are taught how to make the best use of their limbs and how to use various appliances. They like to be independent and should be encouraged to help themselves; watch carefully and give help when required. Some handicapped children may look strange, but when you talk to them, you will find them like other children. Remember that they really look forward to a visit from you.

Some children have jerky movements and cannot use their limbs normally. Others have deformed limbs or no limbs at all. You may need to talk in a loud voice to children who are slightly deaf and you may have to guide children who have poor sight. They all need to feel wanted and loved.

Care of children in wheelchairs

Some children are able to get themselves into their wheelchairs or will tell you what to do to help them. The Australian lift can be used if two people are available and the patient is heavy.

A child who has to sit in a chair will feel cold unless properly dressed and covered adequately. See that the blanket or chair cover does not slip and get tangled in the wheels.

Take care the child does not slip when getting her wheelchair up or down a step or curb.

Put the brake on every time the chair is left unattended.

A child who is confined to a wheelchair likes to be taken out to see people, traffic, the shops and the park.

A few children have electric wheelchairs which, with pressure on a small knob, will travel at a few miles an hour.

Some children, with help, can get from their chairs to the lavatory. Some have to be carried and older ones may have a special handrail and seat fitted so that they can help themselves. A bedpan or urinal can be given to a patient in a wheelchair. You may be asked to help a handicapped child with bathing and washing. This can be done in the bathroom, her bed or even in her chair. Many large towns publish a book for disabled people to tell them where to find lavatories, restaurants, shops and places of entertainment where wheelchairs can be used and special arrangements can be made for them. You should study the Society's booklet "People in Wheelchairs" for further details on this subject.

Care of Children with Artificial Limbs and Calipers (leg irons)

Children are taught how to use these and will know how to put them on. They may ask you to fasten them. Artificial limbs are sometimes powered by batteries.

A child who is paralysed will need:

(a) Special care when dressing. Always put the paralysed or disabled limb into the clothes first. Put your arm through the opposite end of the sleeve or trouser leg and then draw the child's arm or leg towards you to put on the clothes.

(b) Help with feeding. Here you should adopt the same method as for feeding a helpless patient in bed (see p. 33).

Blind children soon learn to feel their way about and like to touch you to get to know you. They like to listen to music, have stories read to them, use swings and climbing frames. Blind children learn to read Braille which consists of a series of raised dots on paper.

Deaf children cannot hear and therefore cannot learn to speak in the same way as other children. They make sounds which they are unable to hear. Partially deaf children often wear hearing aids which help them. Some children lip read, so face the child when speaking so that he can see your lip movements — speak slowly and clearly. These children like doing things with their hands, such as making models, doing jigsaw puzzles.

The Red Cross runs clubs, camps and other services for disabled people and you can read more about them in the Society's Manual on welfare services and in the pamphlet entitled "Red Cross Services in Hospitals and in the Community".

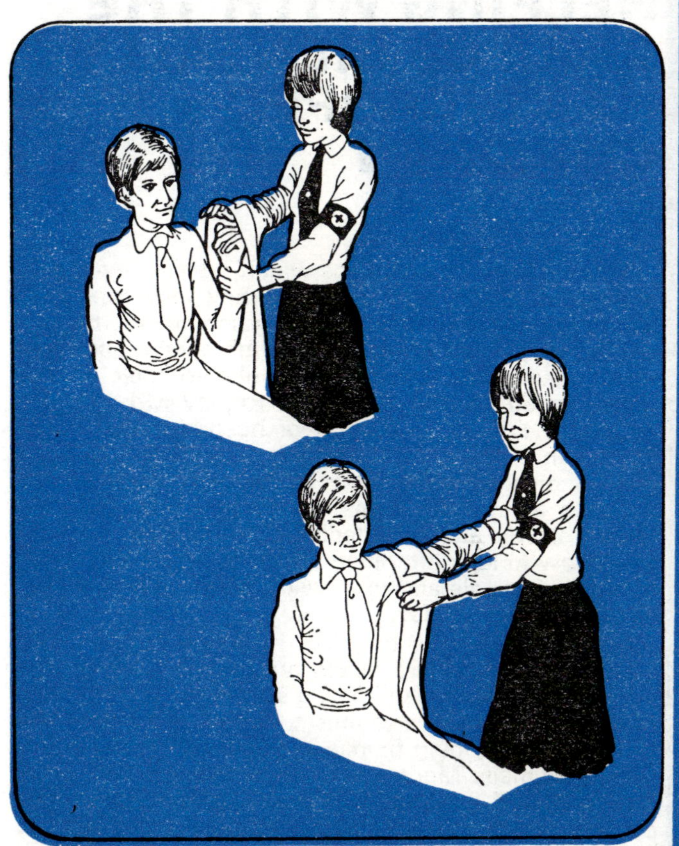

HELPING WITH THE CARE OF MENTALLY HANDICAPPED CHILDREN

Some children have brains which do not develop as quickly as others and therefore they take longer to learn. You can help these mentally handicapped children in many ways. They are most affectionate and will enjoy your company. You may like to look after a handicapped child in a family or to play with children in one of the special homes or hospitals. You could help with a riding or swimming club, teach them to play a musical instrument or accompany them on holidays away from home. Remember they must be taught slowly and repeatedly. This includes teaching them how to look after themselves, to wash and dress, to eat their meals and to develop good table manners as well as how to play.

Like most children they like to play with sand and water, with cardboard boxes and empty plastic containers. They often learn to sing simple songs and many of them love to move to music. Out of doors they like swings and climbing frames, picking wild flowers and seeing animals. Mentally handicapped children often lead sheltered lives and so do not understand all the dangers which you will know. You must remember this and take great care when with them. For instance, if you take one of them out for a walk, until she has been taught kerbside drill, take her hand in yours and hold it firmly when traffic is about and when you are crossing roads.

HELPING WITH THE CARE OF THE AGED

As people grow old the body gradually "wears out" and does not function as well as it used to. Because of this many old people cannot move very well and some are confined to their homes. Others go to live in homes for old people or in flatlets specially arranged for them to live in so that they have each other's company.

You will find that some old people have outlived all their friends, and if their families have moved away from them they will be very lonely.

This problem of loneliness in old age is one of the greatest of our time and one which is as yet unsolved. It is very difficult for most of us to imagine what it would be like to go for days without speaking to anyone.

Although the services of statutory authorities and voluntary organisations are available, often what the elderly need is a regular visit from someone with time to listen. Even when members from the social services call upon them, there are long periods of the day when they have little to do and no one to talk to. A common characteristic of old people is their independence, and you will have to be very tactful if you want to help them.

The first step is to show an interest in them. You may meet with rebuff or brusqueness at first. Some old people who have lived alone for some time will react in this way. You must also be aware that there will be some days when they do not want companionship, when they are in pain or just wish to be left alone. Respect this desire and return another day.

If you are lucky enough to establish a friendship, foster it by constant attention. To be unreliable is worse than not helping at all. If you promise to visit or to do a job, you must never let them down. If you are ill yourself get someone else to take your place. This is one of the great advantages of belonging to an organisation such as the Red Cross — there will always be someone to take over for you.

Once you have been accepted as a friend — and a reliable one — there will be many things you can do. First it is important to use the correct form of address. Always call old people by their names — Mrs. Green or Mr. Brown — unless they ask you to do otherwise.

As you will know, it is sometimes difficult to keep warm in very cold weather, and this is especially so if you cannot move around very much, or are able to move only slowly. It is absolutely essential for old people to keep warm (see p. 23) and you can help to achieve this by visiting to make up the fire, to see that they are able to put on enough warm clothes, and that they have enough food and warm drinks. Ask about errands when you visit. There may be shopping to be done, a letter to be posted or a prescription to take to the chemist. When you shop, remember that some old people have little or nothing above their retirement pension. This has to pay for light, heat, clothes as well as food.

Financial help can be given in the form of "supplementary pension" through the Social Security service but many people refuse to apply for this, believing it to be 'charity'. If you are asked to collect the pension for your friend, realise that this is a privilege entrusted to you and go to the Post Office for it as soon as you can. Living on a tight budget, your friend will not be able to wait for days beyond the date it is due to her. This budget influences the shopping you do. Do not buy the most expensive cuts of meat but, remembering food values, buy those which she can afford, and make certain that you buy food she likes.

You may feel able to do a little cooking (see p. 34), make tea or heat soup when you visit. If there is a garden, notice whether it needs weeding or the grass needs cutting. If you change library books remember that your friend will, in all probability, have tastes different from yours. Ask her whether she likes novels, biographies, travel books, etc. Here again it is of the utmost importance that your help is regular. No matter how busy you are your friend must know for certain that you will appear at the time or on the day you have promised.

If your adopted old person is deaf, speak slowly and distinctly so she is able to watch your lips. If her fingers are no longer nimble, she may need help with cutting her finger nails, doing up buttons or opening a tin of meat for her cat or dog.

If her sight is impaired and she is trying to do some sewing, leave several needles threaded for her to use between your visits. Libraries have books with large print which she may find easier to read, and for registered blind people there are special facilities such as the Nuffield Talking Book Library.

You can help by compiling a library list or by posting recorded tapes. The form of your help must be influenced by what she can do, and by her interests, and you should try to think of ways to help which are based on her individual needs.

Lastly remember that all friendships are two-way and your friend will want to give as well as to receive. You may find that she is able to teach you or help you with things you cannot do, such as embroidery or tapestry work, or (if a man) with carpentry or fly-tying, etc. Accept graciously if you are offered small gifts such as sweets or a treasure from the past. Your pleasure as well as your help will give happiness.

HELPING WITH THE CARE OF PEOPLE HOME FROM HOSPITAL

When people return home from being ill or from having an operation in hospital they often do not feel as well as they had expected to be. Getting out of bed, dressing and the journey home, together with the excitement about leaving hospital, make them tired and sometimes weaker than they had anticipated.

If you know someone who has just been discharged from hospital there may be several ways in which you can be of help. For instance if it is your mother, you will be able to help her with your brothers and sisters, with getting the table ready for meals, helping with the washing up, bedmaking, shopping and washing.

Try to do personal services too. Some days suggest she stays in bed late and give her breakfast there, or give her a supper tray so that she can go to bed early. If she has a plaster on a broken arm she may need help in doing her hair, dressing and cooking.

If the patient lives alone or is elderly she will particularly welcome your visit. Again it may be errands to run, a coal scuttle to be filled, shopping or medicines to be collected, a garden bed to be weeded or a simple meal to prepare (see p. 34). Mothers with young children would probably welcome having them taken away for play for a short time. Remember to adapt your help to the patient's individual needs and interests. Always it is the constancy of your help which is important. If you 'adopt' someone like this, ask one of your friends to take over when you go on holiday until the patient is quite well and fully recovered. Presents are not necessary but a small bunch of wild or garden flowers are welcomed by most people and a home-made cake or home-grown vegetables would be much appreciated.

Appendix—Summary of Infectious Diseases

(*not for examination purposes*)

Disease	*Signs and Symptoms*	*Nursing*
Chickenpox	Rise of temperature. Rash on trunk, face, scalp and limbs. Spots turning to blisters and scabs.	Isolate. Prevent scratching. Keep the skin clean. Apply calamine lotion.
Gastro-enteritis.	Vomiting. Diarrhoea. Abdominal pain.	Isolate. Give plenty of water to drink.
German measles (Rubella)	Slight rise of temperature. Small pink spots which run together appear on the face and spread downwards. Swelling of neck glands.	Bedrest during period of pyrexia (raised temperature). Light or full diet.
Influenza	Rise of temperature. Sore throat, hoarseness of voice, nasal discharge, cough and headache.	Isolate. Bedrest during period of pyrexia. Give plenty of fluids.
Measles	Nasal discharge, eyes sore and watering, cough. Rise of temperature. White spots inside mouth, then a deep red blotchy rash on the face, spreading downwards.	Isolate. Bedrest during period of pyrexia. Clean eyes and mouth. Give plenty of fluids and a light diet.
Mumps	Rise of temperature. Stiff neck and jaw. Earache. Swelling and pain of gland in front of ear.	Isolate and give semi-solids to eat. Avoid strongly flavoured food.
Whooping Cough	Cough which occurs in spasms and may end in a 'whoop'. Sometimes vomiting after coughing.	Give food and fluid after a spasm of coughing with vomiting.

YOUTH NURSING SYLLABUS

The syllabus must consist of a minimum total of 16 hours instruction which may be increased as required. The Course consists of 11 sessions as shown in the following syllabus. Where it is considered that the age and ability of the students enables them to absorb longer training sessions, the syllabus may be given in 10 sessions. In no circumstances may fewer than 10 sessions be given and the minimum total of 16 hours must not be reduced. The minimum age for candidates is 11 years.

Session 1

Introduction and Discussion

Helping to care for the patient
The Sickroom (suggest students should draw plans and make models)

Demonstration and Practice

The principles of bedmaking
Preparing a bed for a patient
Putting a patient into bed

Session 2

Making a patient comfortable in bed
Changing a top sheet
Moving a patient; turning and lifting a patient

Session 3

Making a bed with a patient in it; changing a drawsheet and a bottom sheet
Getting a patient out of bed and making her comfortable in a chair

Session 4

Aids to a patient's comfort in bed
Care of pressure areas
Care of the hair, mouth and teeth

Session 5

Care of the skin and nails
Helping to bath a patient in the bathroom; bathing a patient in bed

Session 6

Observation of the patient - clinical observations
Taking the temperature - by mouth; in the axilla
Counting the pulse and respiration rates

Session 7

Attending to the needs of the patient
Care of the patient when vomiting
Use of bedpans and urinals

Session 8

The patient's diet - a balanced diet
Special diets - light diet; fluid diet
Serving meals; feeding a patient
Making drinks

Session 9

The patient's medicines - care of medicines
Giving a medicine in liquid or solid form
Prevention of accidents

Session 10

Care of wounds; sterilisation
Treating minor injuries - cuts and scratches

Session 11

Revision

YOUTH NURSING SYLLABUS

A minimum total of 11 hours instruction which may be increased as required. The Course consists of 7 sessions. In no circumstances may fewer than 7 sessions be given and the minimum total of 11 hours must not be reduced. The minimum age is 13 years.

Session 1

Revision of care and comfort of a patient in bed - bedmaking
Revision of giving medicines
Giving of inhalations

Session 2

Revision of care and comfort of a patient in bed (cont.)
Observation of patient - revision of taking temperature, pulse and respiration rates
Using temperature charts
Treatment of inflammation - general treatment; local treatment - applying a Kaolin poultice; applying a cold compress

Session 3

Helping with the care of an infectious patient
Prevention of spread of infection
Prevention of infection by immunity
Revision of patient's toilet - care of skin, nails, hair and mouth

Session 4

Washing a patient's hair in bed
Treating infested hair
Helping with the care of a sick or convalescent child
Revision of attending to needs of a patient - vomiting; use of bedpans and urinals

Session 5

Care of physically handicapped children - lifting and dressing; children in wheelchairs and with artificial limbs and calipers
Feeding a helpless patient
Helping blind, deaf and mentally handicapped children

Session 6

Helping with the care of the aged
Revision of bedmaking - changing bottom sheet and drawsheet; aids to comfort; care of pressure areas
Revision of diets, with special reference to the aged

Session 7

Helping with the care of people home from hospital
Revision of care of wounds and bandaging
Revision of prevention of accidents

INTRODUCTORY NURSING COURSE

This course is intended for those who wish to acquire the nursing skills which are needed for the care of the family in the home. The instruction is mainly practical with simple theory to explain the underlying reasons for the various procedures and methods used.

There is no examination but Attendance Vouchers may be issued to those who attend the full course.

Text Book

Practical Nursing Manual of The British Red Cross Society, current edition.

Qualifications of Lecturers

Registered Sick Children's Nurse
State Registered Nurse
State Enrolled Nurse
B.R.C.S. Instructor

Guide to Lecturers

The course should consist of a minimum of four sessions of 1½-2 hours each. Suitable equipment must be made available at each session for students to undertake practical work, but as the emphasis of the course is on "home" nursing, equipment normally found in the home should be used wherever possible. The Lecturer may have the assistance of a Demonstrator.

Syllabus

Session 1

Introduction

The Sickroom - furniture, heating, lighting and ventilation
Equipment - improvisation of equipment
Principles of bedmaking - preparing a bed for a patient - helping a patient into bed

Session 2

Bedmaking continued -

Aids to comfort in bed - changing top, bottom and drawsheets - making a bed with patient in it
Moving a patient - in bed - out of bed and into a chair - into a wheelchair (for further guidance on the handling of patients in wheelchairs see The British Red Cross Society Handbook, *People in Wheelchairs, Hints for Helpers*)

Session 3

Patient's toilet - bathing in the bathroom - bathing in bed
Care of mouth, hair, nails, skin
Care of pressure areas
Care when vomiting
Giving a bedpan or urinal
Observations
Giving medicines
Routine of a patient's day

Session 4

Patient's diet - preparation of meals and drinks - feeding a patient
Care of - the infectious patient; the sick child; the elderly patient; the physically or mentally handicapped patient; the patient home from hospital